TOP
TUNG
ACUPUNCTURE POINTS

Also by Brad Whisnant and Deborah Bleecker:

Mastering Tung Acupuncture, Distal Imaging for Fast Pain Relief, 2nd edition
Pain Case Studies with Distal Acupuncture, a Week in a Tung Clinic
Pain Case Studies with Distal Acupuncture, Volume Two
Treat Back Pain Distally

TOP
TUNG
ACUPUNCTURE POINTS

_____

CLINICAL HANDBOOK

BRAD WHISNANT, LAC, DAOM
DEBORAH BLEECKER, LAC, MSOM

Copyright © 2015 by Deborah Bleecker and Brad Whisnant
1st Edition
Draycott Publishing, LLC

The author of this book does not dispense medical advice or prescribe the use of any technique as a form of treatment for physical, emotional, or medical problems without the advice of a physician, either directly or indirectly. The intent of the author is only to offer information of a general nature to help you in your quest for emotional and spiritual well-being. In the event you use any of the information in this book for yourself, which is your constitutional right, the author and the publisher assume no responsibility for your actions.

Every effort has been made to make this book as complete and as accurate as possible. However, there may be mistakes both typographical and in content. Therefore, this text should be used only as a general guide and not as the ultimate source of information.

ISBN-13:978-1-940146-13-3

CONTENTS

INTRODUCTION

It is almost futile to write a book about Tung acupuncture. Words cannot describe how amazing the points are, and the richness of the underlying theory. Books need to be written to spread the word and communicate with others, and books are a great starting point. If you have read any of our books prior to this one, or have been to one of my seminars, you will hear me preach.

I can only show you the path, it is you who must walk it. Our parents can guide us in life, but it is up to us to live it! We can talk about love, we can define love, but love can only be truly experienced by embracing a loved one, or seeing the sunset over an ocean, or staring into the eyes of your child. Love must be experienced to be truly understood. Tung points, and more correctly, the practice of medicine, can only be understood through practice.

It is only after giving thousands of treatments that we can start to form an opinion. It is only then that we can start to form a judgment about a principle, a theory, or a treatment plan. It is this experience that our industry desperately needs.

Experience is what you got by not having it when you need it. ~Author Unknown

We need scholars of treatments, who are in the trenches treating day in and out, not more scholars of books, or "paper tiger" theorists. This book was written for the medical provider who is ready to treat, ready to roll her sleeves up, treat patients, learn and fail, and continue to study. My ultimate hope is that this book guides you to form your own opinions that differ from mine.

"Well done is better than well said"
Benjamin Franklin

My reality is not your reality. Your life is not my life. We all start on a path, and then we diverge and walk our own paths. Our differences should be celebrated, not mocked. Our measuring stick should be the health and healing we can deliver to our patients. It is not by theory, but in actual healing, and actual medical experience. Our theories are the first step. However, the clinic, our patient, and the treatment itself is where you and I *must* walk the path. Our path is not to talk about it, not to think about it, not to theorize or bicker, but to treat! This book is for those people. I hope you enjoy it.

This book does *not* include all the Tung points. Just as a conversation you have every day does not include every word in the English language. I have included the points I use every day in my clinic. These are the points I have used for over 60,000 treatments, and over seven years. I have used all the Tung points, but the question is, which points do you use the most? Depending on your own personal style, your patients, your strengths, and your attitude, you will develop your favorite theories and points.

I have also attempted to present a fair number of points to treat each issue. You might ask why I included 33.01, 33.02, and 33.03, but not 66.13, 66.14, and 66.15? These points treat similar issues. There is also a famous point for fatigue, 1010.22, which is Bi Yi. I did not include this point because 77.08 is a better point. It is a better point because most patients prefer to be needled in the area of ST 36, rather than the side of their nose.

Why did I not include 77.09, a famous Tung for shoulder pain? Because we have included Fan Hou Jue. Even if we had included Fan Hou Jue, 77.09 is very close to ST 38. We already know from TCM School that ST 38 or 77.09 is great for shoulder pain.

The biggest difference you will notice is that in this book, we have included Zang Fu diagnosis terminology. This will certainly be a controversial idea. The reason we did this is that when you go to TCM school, you learn the language of Chinese medicine. Ninety nine percent of us went to TCM School. One of the hardest things for TCM people to do when they are first learning Tung points is to understand the theory behind the points.

Master Tung spoke in Western medical terms. He was quoted as explaining that the reason for this is that Western medical terms were more accepted during his time. This does not mean that he used a Western medical diagnosis. His theory, which is a family theory, dates back 2,000 years. The Tung system has many theories, but the root of it is the diagnosis of the Five Zang organs.

Master Tung diagnosed disease as disorders of the Five Zang organs, the LU, HT, SP, KD, and the LV. If any of the Five Zang were diseased, the body could not be healthy. He further separated all diseases as either a Qi disease, or a blood disease. That is the secret of diagnosing in a Tung way. Master Tung diagnosed this way, yet he communicated in Western terms.

This can be confusing if all you see for back pain treatments is not the terms Qi and blood stagnation with LV and KD deficiency or excess, but you see lower back pain with osteophytes, compression, and stenosis. The first question is which part of the lower back is affected? Where are the osteophytes located, and how much stenosis, and compression are there? We do not diagnose in Western terms. We treat the branch, but we also treat the root.

It is not a secret that Master Tung did not give theory to his students. When people asked him about specific points, he repeatedly told them to "observe for yourself, and think about it." You can see why over the years so many different Tung disciples have come up with different ideas or theories, since most of them were left to their own devices to theorize the functions of the points. To me it is irrelevant. Tung points work, regardless of which theory is applied to them. My personal spin is from my two teachers, Dr. Wei Chieh Young, and Dr. Tan. You will see both of their teachings in my words.

Regardless of the theory you use, these points are like gravity. Gravity works whether you think you understand it or not. These points also work, even if you do not know why you are using them. Your clinical success will improve if you understand the reasons why the points work. However, anyone can insert Ling Gu and get results for lower back pain.

We have added the Zang Fu indications to the Tung points, for the first time. This will help the reader to understand how to use these points. An example of this is headaches. There are so many points that treat headaches. You can just choose a Tung point, and use it to treat headaches. That is why so many people say that sometimes they use Tung points and they are amazing, and other times they do not work so well. It is because they are not treating the root correctly.

A headache can be caused by so many things. It can be caused by any of the Five Zang, Six Fu, wind, damp, heat, cold, stagnation, excess, phlegm, and the list is endless. We must choose the correct point to treat the condition correctly. That is why I have included a Zang Fu diagnosis. This is the language of 99% of TCM acupuncturists. We have also included the classical indications, so you can see how these TCM diagnoses manifest as Western complaints.

I also think it was necessary because Western medical terms get increasingly specific. I often receive e-mails from acupuncturists asking me if a specific Tung point can be used to treat lockjaw, when it is indicated to treat TMJ. They want to know if the point will work for something other than the indications listed. They will also ask if a point will treat osteoarthritis, when the point is just indicated for arthritis. This is a Western term, and it shows how we need to acknowledge and understand Western terms, just as in Tung's time Western terms were more used. However, we must know the root cause! We must treat the disease, that is the secret.

The secret is using 88.12, 88.13, and 88.14, which are on the liver channel, to treat a headache that is caused by fatigue, when the diagnosis is a weak liver. It is not to say that "Da Bai, point 22.04, is indicated for headaches, let's try that." In which case you would hold your breath, close your eyes, and say that it must work, because my book says it treats headaches. We have to ask why? We need to diagnose, however you do that, to find the root pathology.

We have focused primarily on modern diseases. Master Tung saw more polio, rheumatic fever, scarlet fever, mumps, and tuberculosis (which is why there are more points for these), than tight upper back muscles, and pain at the area of GB 21, and TW 15, that we see so often in modern clinics.

Do you know why Master Tung has so few points to treat stress and insomnia? It is because he did not see it that much. He also has more points for polio than for stress, because polio was more common. This is not common in America, but I have treated it in Vietnam, India, Honduras, and Guatemala. These countries have different diseases than we do. Our culture, diet, and income levels affect which diseases we get.

I have never treated dry cholera in America. That is caused by poor sanitation, parasites, and microbes in our water and food. I have treated it in rural India, and rural Vietnam. There are also not a lot of points to treat insomnia. The reason for that is that the people he treated were non postindustrial people, like we have in America.

Most non postindustrial culture people who work hard all day, do not have sleep disorders. They are exhausted at the end of the day. In America, where we do not exercise as much, and we are continually stimulated by food, our IPad, TV screens, too much stress, never winding down, checking e-mail in bed, or Facebook in bed at 11 pm, of course we have more sleep problems than they do in rural India, where they pick rice all day in the fields.

I have omitted many points, because they focus on diseases which we do not have in our culture any more, or the ones we do not see in acupuncture clinics. If someone has scarlet fever, he would go to the emergency room, not to an acupuncturist. Master Tung also did not have any points to treat Type 2 diabetes, because it did not exist back then. We do have points that harmonize the spleen and stomach, and treat the spleen or pancreas, but the indication of Type 2 diabetes is an extrapolation of the original Tung indication, that never mentioned diabetes.

Dao Ma Theory

Another focus of this book is the Dao Ma concept, because your success will increase exponentially when you treat in this fashion. Once you are amazing and people call you Dr. Jesus, then you can just insert one needle in one magical point and get great results. Until you can do that, do your patient a favor, and treat in a Dao Ma fashion. Use either two or three points together. This is what Master Tung did, and I would suggest that after his 500,000 treatments, he was still using the Dao Ma technique, then we should also.

The Dao Ma Needling Technique of Master Tung Ching-Chang, was one of the clinical methods he most frequently employed. This technique can succinctly be stated as follows: three points are needled simultaneously to profoundly 'obtain qi' (De Qi) and rapidly effect a cure. Dr. Tung did not greatly concern himself with 'supplementing' (Bu) or 'draining' (Xie) needle techniques, but rather with powerfully 'obtaining qi' (De Qi) to influence the 'Reaction Areas' of the points needled. In this style of acupuncture, the more you obtain the qi, the quicker you got results. (Master Tung's lecture on Acupuncture) *Advanced Tung Style Acupuncture Dr. Maher*

Reaction Area

Treating the reaction area is the secret of treating the five Zang organs. It is also a deeper understanding of Tung acupuncture. It explains why both 44.06 and 22.05 treat fatigue. The reaction area of 44.06 is the heart, whereas the reaction area of 22.05 is the lung. This helps you choose your points, depending on which Zang is affected.

"A reaction area is neurophysical acupuncture. This reflects the knowledge of the delicate energy of the body and the neuroanatomical and neurophysiologic aspects of the body. This acupuncture style also corrects and heals the body through the manipulation of the peripheral and central nervous system by affecting the neuraxis, the actual anatomy, physiology and pathophysiology of the body. (Advanced Tung Style Acupuncture Dr. Maher)"

In this book, we have in some cases omitted the depth of the needle insertion. Master Tung and his disciples all say that the most important thing to consider about a point is not the depth, nor the location, nor the theory, but to elicit a "Qi response." Master Tung said "the faster we can bring Qi to the point, the faster we can heal disease."

This emphasis on getting the Qi, does not mean to "kill the patient and put them through the roof with your needle." What it does mean is to get a sensation that can be as mild as a gentle muscle grab on the needle. The depth at which Qi arrives is not specific to the point, but to your patient. We have patients who are underweight, overweight, very muscular, bloated with water retention, and who have too much inflammation. All these things will affect the needle depth. I don't think it is practical to say that we should needle 77.08 half a cun for knee pain, one cun for stomach problems, and two cun for head problems. If our patient has large legs, or very thin legs, the insertion depth needs to be adjusted.

It seems impractical to say that Ling Gu and Da Bai have an insertion depth of .5 to 1 cun. An example of this is my grandmother, she is 96, and her Yang Qi is sinking. She needs energy. The Qi sensation arrived at .25 cun. Should I continue to insert the needle to a predetermined depth? I don't think so. The depth of any needle is where the Qi arrives.

Most points have Pin Yin names and numbers. Some points only have names, like Fan Hou Jue. The regions of 22, 77, and 88 were the most commonly used by Master Tung to treat chronic diseases. For acute diseases, the regions of 11 and 1010 were used most.

He used points on the regions of 44 and 55 least often, according to his disciples. I have included a general overview of the Master Tung ear points. I did not include a lot of ear points, because I prefer to use Auricular acupuncture vs. Tung ear points. I did not include points on the torso, because those points are not needled, they are only bled.

Finger Regions

All of the regions are pretty straightforward, except the fingers. The fingers have "lines" on them. The lines are the A, B, C, D, E, F, G, and H lines. If you look at your index finger, with the palm facing you, the A line would be where the pink and white skin meet, which is on the lateral side of your finger.

The C line is on the midline of the index finger. If you continue around your index finger, where the pink and white skin meet is the E line. If you continue around the index finger to the dorsal side, the midline of the finger is the G line. If you were to continue around your finger, you would end up back at the A line, where the dorsal white skin meets the palmar side pink skin.

Now that you know where the A, C, E, and G lines are, the B, D, F, H are between the other lines. I know it sounds a little confusing, but once you start to see the eight lines that run down your fingers it's very easy to understand.

The last tricky part of the finger points are the points with multiple points. An example of this is 11.27, which is a five point unit. Another example is 11.17, which is a two point unit. The way these points are treated is by needling the points as separated into equidistant locations. For example, 11.17 is on the D line, between the PIP joint and the MIP joint of the index finger. Point 11.17 has two points. These two points are equidistant on the D line, between the PIP and MIP joint. If you were to look at the index finger, between the PIP and MIP joint, you would see three equal sections.

Wu Hu - Five Tigers   Mu - Wood Point

Consider 11.27, it is a five point unit on the thumb joint shaft, between the PIP and DIP joint. The metacarpal shaft is equally divided by five points that comprise the 11.27 five point unit. The fingers are not meant to be confusing, and if you go slowly in the beginning, it is not as hard as it sounds.

Ultimately, this book is a guide for the modern day Western clinic. We see physical, emotional, spiritual, acute, chronic, easy, and difficult patients. We also see patients who will only give us one shot before they quit coming in, and some patients will let us treat them 30 times and let us treat all sorts of ailments. It is good for our modern patients who need to have acupuncture proven to them. It works great for patients who are sensitive to needles, and those that don't care and just want to get better.

This book cuts through all the fat, and gets to the meat. As I am sure Master Tung would say to me if I were talking to him right now, "just sit with these points, use what you need, understand and think about what you don't know, understand their usefulness, and their limitations. Keep what you need, and let go of what does not serve you."

This book is focused on how we treat in modern clinics every day. This is what my clinic has looked like over the last seven years, and specifically the last three years and 22,000 treatments.

The top complaints, which is about 95% of all cases are:

- Upper neck/shoulder
- Low back
- Pain anywhere
- Sciatica
- Joint pain, knee, elbow, fingers toes, and shoulder
- Headache, trigeminal neuralgia, TMJ jaw pain
- Sleep (too much or too little)
- Digestive disorders such as IBS, Crohn's disease, bloating, gas, constipation, and diarrhea
- Stress/depression/anxiety/fatigue/libido/no zest for life
- The big three, heart issues, Type 2 diabetes, Cholesterol
- Female issues, menstrual, hot flashes etc.
- Allergies and breathing issues
- Fertility (male and female)
- General wellness, neuropathy, numbness, and weird diseases no one else can cure
- Last resort -Alzheimer's, Parkinson's, tinnitus, MS, auto immune etc.

We do treat other ailments, like hypoxemic respiratory failure or scarlet fever, but we do not treat it all the time.

The goal of this book is to help you learn how to quickly use 90% of the points you would normally use in clinic.

In closing, please continue to study. Continue to learn from others. Don't ever stop learning. A wasted day is a day that you do not learn anything. Improvise, overcome, and adapt. Never quit, don't give up, breathe, and relax.

BASICS OF MASTER TUNG NEEDLES

Ashi Locations

There is no need to locate Ashi points. You can use Ashi locations if you choose to, but the locations of the Tung points don't require a point to be Ashi. Sometimes I will locate the Tung point, and *then* locate the Ashi point around it, but it is not necessary. The point will still be effective even if there is no Ashi sensation.

Needle Size

You can use any size or brand you like. I use 36 gauge. I know some acupuncturists who use 28 gauge, and some who use 40 gauge. They all work. You do not need to tonify, sedate, rotate, or flick. There is no needle manipulation in the Tung system. Insert your needles and relax. Make sure your needles are not flopping around, but you don't need to needle deeply either. Most points are inserted .25-.50 cun on the arms, legs are .5-1.5 cun, the fingers and head are about .1-.3 cun.

Internal Medicine

Although Americans only seek acupuncture for pain relief, Master Tung acupuncture is also very effective for internal problems. Many points also address the root, when they treat the manifestation.

Needle Retention

The cycle of Qi is about 28 minutes. We also know from MRI studies that the brain will respond well for about 28.8 minutes. I have my patients sit or lie down for 25 to 30 minutes.

Number of Needles Used

We should always try to limit our needles. However, do not insert a few needles and leave your patient without determining you have complete pain relief. You should use as few needles as possible, but as many as necessary.

Expectation of Results

You should expect a 90-100% reduction in the pain while your patient is lying on the treatment table. I expect this for at least 85% of my patients. Of the remaining patients, 5% do net get relief, and 10% have a 25-75% reduction in pain while on the treatment table.

Most of my patients come in once a week. I treat about 100 patients per week. Only 16 of those come twice a week. Not all patients need two treatments a week. There are many factors that determine the frequency of treatments.

I try to treat all my patients three to four times before we make a final judgment about whether acupuncture will work for their condition. This does not always work. Some people do not come back, and some people only get one or two treatments. We usually expect instant pain relief. However, I always advise patients to allow three to four visits over a ten-day period to see if it will work for them. We will then decide what further treatment is necessary.

Opposite Side Treatment
Most points are treated on the opposite side of the pain. If you are in doubt, treat the opposite side. There are some theories that require a same side insertion.

Having the Patients Move during Treatment
Insert the needles and ask the patient to recreate the pain. You will know within 1-2 seconds if they feel better. If they *cannot move* while on the table, or recreate the pain, just treat it as if it were there, right now. You can have the patient recreate the pain after the treatment.

Efficacy
I appreciate the fact that Master Tung acupuncture is straightforward. You insert the needles, breathe, and heal. That is it! There are no tricks, no magic, no guessing, and no hoping that you relieved the pain. You know it immediately. It is easy, safe, reliable, consistent, and effective acupuncture.

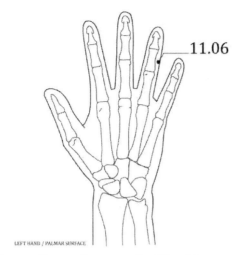

11.06

11.06
Huan Chao
Return to the Nest

Palmar side

Huan Chao - Return To The Nest

TCM FUNCTIONS

This point regulates the San Jiao, which regulates Qi disorders. It invigorates Kidney essence, tonifies the Liver and Kidneys. It moves Liver Qi and blood stagnation, harmonizes the Liver, and disperses Liver Qi.

REACTION AREA

Liver, Kidney

LOCATION AND NEEDLE TECHNIQUE

On the ulnar side of the middle segment of the ring finger, in the center between the 2nd and 3rd finger creases. Perpendicular insertion where the white and pink skin meet, on the E line. Tap the bone to activate the Kidney indications.

You can also needle a second 11.06 point, this could be called 11.06 A. This point is on the same finger, but on the A line. This point is less frequently used, but can be used as an adjunct point if needed.

CLASSICAL INDICATIONS

Symptoms that can be treated with these points include: uterine pain, uterine tumor, and uterine inflammation, and irregular menstruation, leucorrhea with reddish discharge, tubal obstruction, uterine retroversion, frequent urination, vaginal swelling, and frequent miscarriage.

11.06
Huan Chao
Return to the Nest

CLINICAL APPLICATIONS

Please refer to 11.24. Points 11.06 and 11.24 are always used together in the treatment of infertility. They are the first choice to treat infertility, since most infertility patients have Kidney and Liver issues. However, treat infertility according to the TCM diagnosis. These points don't treat "infertility." They treat infertility when a patient has infertility caused by Liver, Kidney or other issues with the uterus.

Point 11.06 is the LV and KD reaction area, and 11.24 is the reaction area of the uterus. If a patient has infertility due to these reasons, these two points are remarkably effective to treat it. If a patient has infertility due to another pathology, which does not involve the Liver, Kidneys, or uterus, these points are not a good choice.

I always combine 11.24 with 11.06. Many people say to treat these points on the right side, since women are treated on the right side, and men are treated on the left side. Clinically that is an option, however I prefer to use alternate sides for each treatment.

Point 11.06 focuses on regulating the San Jiao, and communicating with the Kidney. Since these points are on the ring finger, the fourth finger in the Tung system is the Liver. These points and this finger will communicate with the Liver.

In my experience, if the correct pattern identification is used, and the correct treatment points, infertility can be cured in more than 75% of all couples, using acupuncture alone. I always treat both partners.

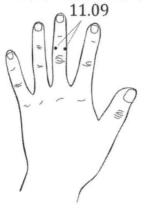

Xin Xi - Heart Knee
11.09

11.09
Xin Xi
Heart Knee

TCM FUNCTIONS
These points have the actions of soothing the liver, moving Qi, and tonifying the kidneys when they are needled close to the bone and through the tendons and small hand muscles.

UPPER JIAO
Nourishes the heart, quickens the blood, transforms stasis and relieves pain.

REACTION AREA
Heart

LOCATION AND NEEDLE TECHNIQUE
Perpendicular insertion on the F and H lines. Grab the finger in the area of the points, and let go. After you let go, insert the needle. Located on both sides of the middle segment of the middle finger on the dorsal side, in the center between the second and third finger creases.

CLASSICAL INDICATIONS
Knee pain and scapula pain, problems closer to the upper spine.

CLINICAL APPLICATIONS
This point is not famous in the West to treat upper back pain, it is the point of choice in Taiwan, where Master Tung lived and practiced, for upper neck and back pain.

Knee pain is the most common indication for this point in the West. It is better for knee pain due to circulation issues, patellar tendonitis, or ST channel knee pain. These points are on the PC channel, and the PC treats the ST channel. The ST channel runs through the knee. Although these points will treat all types of knee pain, they are better for the above listed knee conditions.

11.09
Xin Xi
Heart Knee

A common question is why there is such a strong relationship between the heart and the knee in Tung acupuncture. In my opinion, I believe that the majority of Master Tung's patients were physically active in their jobs. These types of people get knee pain that is arthritic in nature. Arthritis pain is always worse in the morning, before the circulation is improved with activity. This differentiates arthritic pain from inflammatory pain. Pain that is worse at the end of the day is affected by increased swelling. The PC channel is the physical action of the heart in Chinese medicine, whereas the HT channel is the emotional aspect. The PC channel is used to increase heart pumping activity. That is why these points treat knee pain on the PC channel.

To treat knee pain, always combine 11.09 with 11.13. Point 11.09 can be used alone to treat neck pain, and pain in the area of GB 21, TW 15, and BL 43. However, to treat knee pain it should be combined with 11.13.

Point 11.09 will treat any type of knee pain, but it is most effective for knee pain that is arthritic in nature, on the LV or ST channel, or that has a blood deficiency, blood stagnation, or blood heat pathology as the root.

Other indications include knee pain, scapula pain, and problems close to the upper spine.

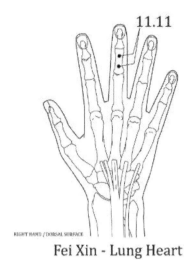

11.11

11.11
Fei Xin
Lung Heart

Fei Xin - Lung Heart

TCM FUNCTIONS
These points move Qi and blood, relieve bone and muscle Bi syndrome, clear the Du channel, and stop pain. They tonify the heart and lung Qi.

REACTION AREA
Heart, Lung

LOCATION AND NEEDLE TECHNIQUE
On the middle segment of the dorsal aspect of the middle finger. Pinch the skin away from the bone, so you have access to more skin. Needle across the bone superficially, towards the little finger. The trick is to pull the skin up, so that the needle does not bury itself into the finger bone.

CLASSICAL INDICATIONS
Common indications are spinal pain, sacral vertebral pain, lumbar pain, neck pain, and calf pain originating in the spine.

CLINICAL APPLICATIONS
These points are excellent for back pain, but there are three distinct differences on what type of back pain. These points are indicated for acute pain. Points on the fingers, the Jing Wells, and Ying Springs are better for acute, fullness, and excess pain, and pain that originates from the spine. The points do treat back muscles and back pain in general, but for the best results, the root cause should be from the bones, spine, or Du channel.

11.11
Fei Xin
Lung Heart

Constriction is also a factor. Another indication is for back pain from a wrenched back. A wrenched back would imply constriction. Since these points are on the PC channel, on the finger, and the middle finger is in the Heart, in the Tung system, would obviously improve blood circulation. This increased circulation will pump blood into a wrenched back. That is why they are effective points to relieve this type of back pain.

We need to be careful with what Western terms we use, they explain conditions but do not tell us the reason why it is that way. A wrenched back can be caused by about 100 different things. We need to treat the root cause, not the symptom of a wrenched back.

In addition, in the Kyoro hand therapy system, the middle finger represents the spine, and these points treat spinal pain on the Du channel. So regardless of which theory you use, these points are valuable to treat acute spine pain on the Du channel, which involves vasoconstriction.

These points are used often to treat acute injuries such as whiplash. They are also useful for patients who have back pain when they get up in the morning. They also treat pain caused by bending over to pick something up, or turning in one direction and suddenly the muscles seize up in the back. They treat acute, traumatic injury of unknown pathologies as well.

These points are also used in another system, which is Su Jok hand therapy. This is a micro hand therapy. It might not make sense why this could treat leg or calf pain, but from Su Jok hand therapy theory, the thumb is the torso, and the index and pinky fingers are the arms. The middle and ring finger are the legs. The trick is that it treats leg and calf pain, but not from any etiology. It only treats calf pain that is caused by spine pain.

When there is compression of the nerves in the spine and back, this causes pain radiation into the calf. These points are used often when patients have a spine or back problem that radiates into the calf. This one point, which is 11.11 and 11.12 are always used together, so I consider them to be one point, can treat the whole problem, the spine, back, bone, and radiation into the calf.

11.11
Fei Xin
Lung Heart

Points 11.11 and 11.12 are always used together. Point 11.11 is used more to treat the upper spine, but it is valuable for any type of spine pain. I would not suggest using 11.11 alone. Always combine it with 11.12, regardless of the location of the spine pain. If you were to try to isolate the area that 11.11 treats, it treats the area of BL 43 at T4.

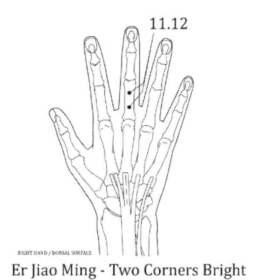

11.12

11.12
Er Jiao Ming
Two Corners Bright

Er Jiao Ming - Two Corners Bright

TCM FUNCTIONS
LOWER JIAO
Move Qi and blood, stop bone and muscle Bi syndrome, clear the Du channel, and stop pain. Invigorate the kidneys, tonify kidney Qi.

UPPER JIAO
Brightens the eyes, dispels damp, and opens the channels and collaterals.

REACTION AREA
Kidney, Eyes

LOCATION AND NEEDLE TECHNIQUE
On the midline of the proximal segment of the middle finger on the dorsal side. Pinch the skin away from the bone, so you have a small amount between your fingers. Needle across the bone, superficially towards the little finger. The trick is to pull the skin up, so your needle does not bury itself into the finger bone. These points are on the G line, and are needled across the middle finger towards the 5th finger.

CLASSICAL INDICATIONS
Sprain in the lumbar region, pain in the supraorbital bone, nasal bone pain, nosebleeds, frontal headaches, eye issues – they brighten the eyes, glaucoma, intraocular eye pressure, and headaches from eye pressure. Other eye indications include, but are not limited to, macular degeneration, vision issues, and floaters.

11.12
Er Jiao Ming
Two Corners Bright

CLINICAL APPLICATIONS

Point 11.12 is always combined with 11.11 to treat pain on the spine. These points are excellent to treat back pain on the Du channel, and there are three distinct differences in the type of back pain. The pain should be acute. It does treat the muscles, but the main function is the bones, or the spine. Point 11.12 is usually for lower back pain, whereas 11.11 is for upper back pain. The PIP joint of the finger is is C1, the MIP joint is C7/T1 and then the knuckle of the hand is usually considered to be L5/S1 in hand acupuncture.

As indicated for 11.11, these points are used for tight muscles. They improve circulation by affecting the heart. When the blood flow to the muscles is improved, the muscles can relax.

Point 11.12 also is used to treat eye problems. It treats eye pain, pressure, wind, redness, fullness, heat, Qi or blood stagnation in the eyes. This is not the first choice to treat eye problems, but they are a nice addition when you want to supplement the other points for the eyes.

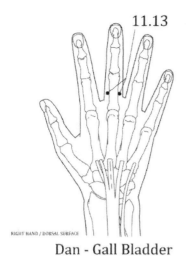

11.13

Dan - Gall Bladder

**11.13
Dan
Gall Bladder**

TCM FUNCTIONS
Tonifies, moves and clears the gallbladder. Nourishes the heart, calms the spirit, and eliminates irritation. It quickens the Qi and blood, transforms stasis, and relieves pain. When needling close to the bone and tendon, we activate the KD and LV tonification.

REACTION AREA
Gallbladder

LOCATION AND NEEDLE TECHNIQUE
In the middle of the proximal segment of the middle finger on the dorsal side. Perpendicular insertion on the F and H line. Hold the finger, as you let go, insert the needle. As you press the points, you are pushing the blood out of the point, it gives you a split second to insert the needle, which makes it less painful for the patient. Insert a half cun needle .1 to .2 cun deep.

CLASSICAL INDICATIONS
Child nightmares, night time crying of babies, and gallbladder dysfunction.

11.13
Dan
Gall Bladder

CLINICAL APPLICATIONS
This point is always used with 11.09 for the treatment of knee pain.

A common question is why there is such a close relationship between the heart and the knee in Tung acupuncture. I would suggest that most of the patients Master Tung treated were people who walked and worked a lot. Typically these types of people get knee pain that is arthritic in nature. Arthritic pain is usually worse in the morning, before we get up and start moving around to improve circulation. Once we start moving around, the pain will usually go away.

This is the difference between arthritic pain that hurts in the morning, when there is poor blood circulation, and the inflammatory type of pain that is worse at the end of the day. It hurts worse because it is swollen from too much movement. Most of Master Tung's patients who had pain, had arthritic type pain. The PC is the physical action of the heart in Chinese medicine, whereas the HT is the emotional center. The PC channel is responsible to get the heart pumping. That explains why these points that are used to treat knee pain are on the PC channel. When this point is used for knee pain, I always combine it with 11.09 and 11.13.

It is also very effective for gallbladder issues, since it is the reaction area of the GB. This is the only time I would use this point alone, without 11.09, is to treat gallbladder issues.

Although an indication often listed for this point is "morbid night crying of babies," most babies do not tolerate being poked in their fingers, and thus I do not use this point for that indication.

The type of palpitations it treats are heart palpitations due to weak heart qi and stagnant liver Qi. I do use this point for people who have nightmares and fear. The middle finger is the PC, and the PC calms the Shen. These points are close to the bone, and thus activate the KD. The KD is responsible for fear.

I have used this point successfully to treat my 4 year old who had awakened with bad dreams. By pressing gently on these points, he was able to calm down and go back to sleep the remainder of the night.

11.13
Dan
Gall Bladder

This point is closer to other Master Tung points on the fingers that are used to treat heart problems, such as palpitations. These points treat heart palpitations because they are on the PC channel on the finger. This is the relationship of the PC and HT, and PC and ST. It is also the reaction area of the GB, which is associated with the HT.

The middle finger is associated with the heart in Tung acupuncture. We know that the PC channel, via TCM theory, is on the middle finger. So the middle finger is responsible for heart issues and conditions. The HT treats the HT, and the PC treats the HT. The PC also treats the ST, via the Zang Fu Bei Tong relationship.

The ST channel runs straight through the heart. The reaction area of this point is the gallbladder, and we know that the GB treats the heart via the Zang Fu Bei Tong theory. That is why these points have a strong connection with the heart. The heart is responsible for emotions, such as joy, in Chinese medicine. This also explains why it treats bad dreams. Bad dreams are a lack of joy.

On a side note, there have been books written about people who have had heart transplants, both mechanical hearts and human hearts. Most of these people report that with a new heart they have the emotions of the person who donated the heart. And people with mechanical hearts report a lack of joy. The research about people who have had both human hearts and mechanical hearts is quite fascinating, and it confirms the beliefs of Chinese medicine from over 3,000 years ago, that the heart is the soul of human beings, not the brain, as Western medicine asserts.

Mu - Wood Point

11.17
Mu
Wood Point

TCM FUNCTIONS

MIDDLE JIAO INDICATIONS
Regulates the middle Jiao, clears liver fire, liver yang rising, moves liver Qi and blood. Harmonizes the liver, and invigorates the kidney.

UPPER JIAO INDICATIONS
Dispels wind and damp, and releases the exterior. Dispels pathogens, brightens the eyes, disperses swelling, resolves pain, calms the Shen, and quiets the spirit.

LOWER JIAO INDICATIONS
Discharges and clears damp heat in the lower Jiao, rectifies Qi in the lower Jiao, removes obstructions from the channels.

REACTION AREA
Liver

LOCATION AND NEEDLE TECHNIQUE
On the medial aspect of the index finger on the palmar side of the line of 0.2 cun away from the midline. These points are on the D line. Perpendicular insertion on the D line. I use a 36 gauge .5 inch needle. Hold the finger firmly, squeeze for a split second, as you release, insert the needle. This point is not painful.

CLASSICAL INDICATIONS
Hyperactivity of Liver Fire and irritability, dry eyes, dry nose, dermatitis of the hands, common cold, stress, anger, crying, stuffy congested nose, sinus issues, respiratory problems, urinary and genital issues, cystitis and hernia. Sweating of the hands, and dermatitis of the hands.

11.17
Mu
Wood Point

CLINICAL APPLICATIONS

Very effective for any nose or eye issue. It treats cold, dry, hot, stuffy, damp or wind, both internal or external issues.

Since there are so few points in the Tung system that are indicated to treat anger, stress, and depression, these are effective for that. I don't use this point alone to treat anger issues. Most patients need to have more issues treated. For this problem, it is helpful to add 1010.01, 1010.05, 1010.06, 1010.08, and 11.17. The points on the head treat the liver to resolve stress. This is a great point combination for patients with stress, anger, and anxiety.

These points can be used for dermatosis and other skin problems. The LI treats the LU, the LU controls the skin, which explains the indications for skin. However, other points are more effective clinically.

These points can be used to treat lower Jiao, urinary, and genital problems. The LI treats the LV and KD, and the image of these points explains the efficacy. They are effective to treat upper rcspiratory problems. The LI treats the LU.

The main indication for these points in the Tung system is for LV fire, and LV stagnation manifesting in patients with anger and stress.

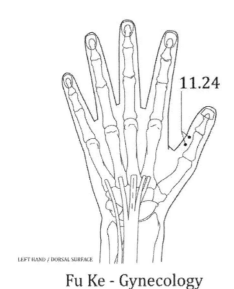

11.24
Fu Ke
Gynecology

Fu Ke - Gynecology

TCM FUNCTIONS
These points supplement, invigorate and regulate the Kidneys and Liver. They move Qi and blood, and regulate the menses. They warm the Palace of the Essence (the uterus), and rectify the lower burner. They dispel cold damp, and eliminate cold in the genitals and lower Jiao.

REACTION AREA
Uterus

LOCATION AND NEEDLE TECHNIQUE
On the ulnar side of the dorsal, proximal segment of the thumb. These points are on the E line. Hold the thumb and press on the area of the points, then release. As you release it, insert the needle. Insert a needle closely along the edge of the phalanx.

The needles are parallel to the thumb, as they slide down next to the bone. This is why they treat the KD and LV, because the needle is inserted through the tendon and is close to the bone. The bone is KD, and the tendon is LV.

CLASSICAL INDICATIONS
Additional indications include: Uterine inflammation, acute or chronic pelvic pain, hysteromyoma, distention of the lower abdomen, female infertility, irregular menstruation, dysmenorrhea, scanty menstruation, fibroids, change the position of the uterus during or after pregnancy, move blood, and or resolve uterine stagnation.

11.24
Fu Ke
Gynecology

CLINICAL APPLICATIONS

These points should be your first choice to treat infertility, because most cases of infertility involve the KD and LV. However, verify that this is the correct pathology. These points do not simply treat infertility. They treat infertility caused by the LV, KD, and uterus.

Point 11.06 is the reaction area of the LV and KD. Point 11.24 is the reaction area of the uterus. If a patient has infertility due to these reasons, these two points are remarkably effective to treat it. If the patient has infertility due to another pathology, that does not involve the LV or KD, or uterus, these points are not a good choice.

I always use 11.24 with 11.06. Although many acupuncturists advise to treat these points on the right side, since they are treating women, I prefer to alternate sides to cover one side for one treatment, and the other side for the next treatment.

These points are also extremely effective to treat all types of uterus issues. Examples of this include menstrual problems, back pain from the menstrual cycle, and headaches caused by irregular hormones. If the female cycle is at the root of the disorder, these points are a good choice.

Clinically these points are a wonderful choice for a mal-positioned uterus or post birth uterus issues, prolapse of the uterus, or back pain stemming from inflammation of the uterus.

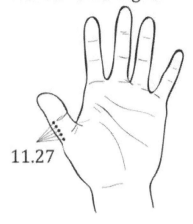

Wu Hu - Five Tigers

11.27
Wu Hu
Five Tigers

TCM FUNCTIONS
Bi syndrome, specifically Damp Bi and Bone Bi. These points clear the channels and collaterals, stop pain, move Qi and blood, and dispel damp.

REACTION AREA
Spleen

LOCATION AND NEEDLE TECHNIQUE
On the radial aspect of the proximal segment of the palmar side of the thumb. Insert the needle on the A line, between the pink and white skin, perpendicular insertion, you must touch the bone. These 5 points are equidistant from each other on the bone. Point 1 starts at the most distal end of the thumb.

CLASSICAL INDICATIONS
Swollen, achy joints, toe pain, gout, sore throat, swollen glands, pneumonia, cough, scrofula. These points are on the LU channel, and the LU treats the throat, osteoarthritis, rheumatoid arthritis, and osteoporosis.

CLINICAL APPLICATIONS
The original indication for Tung was just "treats bone swelling in and throughout the entire body."

These points are used often due to the reaction area, the spleen. It deals with systemic pain and swelling. These points are very useful for autoimmune disorders, they are the top points for this. They treat autoimmune rheumatoid arthritis patients. For these patients points 1-3-5 are chosen for the systemic effects.

11.27
Wu Hu
Five Tigers

This is a five point unit.

Point 1 treats pain of the fingers and wrist, and headaches
Point 2 does not have indications, it is used to assist 1 and 3
Point 3 treats toe pain and headaches
Point 4 treats pain of the dorsal foot and instep
Point 5 treats heel pain

I will frequently use these points for gout, and pain of the big toe. They speed the healing process after a broken toe.

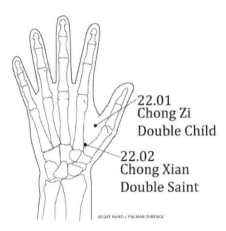

22.01
Chong Zi
Double Child

22.02
Chong Xian
Double Saint

RIGHT HAND / PALMAR SURFACE

22.01
Chong Zi
Double Child

Palmar side

TCM FUNCTIONS
LU channel -Courses the lung, moves Qi and blood, frees channel Qi, and dispels phlegm in the lower Jiao.

BL channel – Dispels wind and dissipates cold, soothes the sinews and quickens the connecting vessels, clears the head and neck, and relieves pain.

REACTION AREA
Lung

LOCATION AND NEEDLE TECHNIQUE
On the thenar eminence, about 1 cun distal to the skin fold, between the first and second metacarpals. Perpendicular insertion.

CLASSICAL INDICATIONS
Back pain, pneumonia, cold and flu, cough, asthma, fibroids, and chest pain.

CLINICAL APPLICATIONS
According to some sources, this will treat GB 21 pain, but I found it is rarely effective for that. This point combination treats a stiff neck, which is also called "fallen pillow syndrome," which is a stiff neck that occurs when you wake up. It is very effective in combination with Ren 24, and GB 39, and/or with 77.01, 77.02, and 77.03. Since it is located close to LU 10, it does have the indications of asthma, flu, and breathing issues. It is clinically useful for this.

22.01
Chong Zi
Double Child

Point 22.01 is considered to be more useful for neck pain, while 22.02 is better for upper back and shoulder pain. These points work best when combined, and are most effective for pain in the area of C1-7 and T1. I would not use them for GB 21 or TW 15 pain, unless the pain in that area is originating from the spine and radiating to that area. It is great for stiff neck. It is not great for a tight upper back that is common in Western patients.

These points are on the LU channel, and they influence the BL, LI, and SP, which explains many of the indications.

I rarely use 22.01 alone, I would suggest you always combine 22.01 with 22.02. These are some of the more popular Tung points, and I would suggest they are not as effective as commonly believed. I do like them, but I would not use these points unless other points were not available. It is relevant we understand these points, but it is clinically more relevant to realize what they do not treat, and their shortcomings.

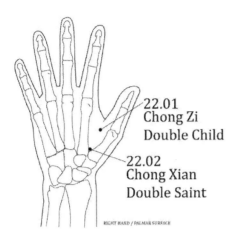

22.01
Chong Zi
Double Child

22.02
Chong Xian
Double Saint

RIGHT HAND / PALMAR SURFACE

22.02
Chong Xian
Double Saint

(Double Immortal)

Palmar

TCM FUNCTIONS
LU channel – courses the lung, moves Qi and blood, frees channel Qi, and dispels damp phlegm in the upper Jiao.

BL channel – dispels wind, dissipates cold, soothes the sinews, and quickens the connecting vessels, clears the head and neck, and relieves pain.

REACTION AREA
Lung, Heart

LOCATION AND NEEDLE TECHNIQUE
The point is located between the first and second metacarpal bones, 2 cun from the skin fold, across from and communicating with Ling Gu (22.05) on the dorsal side of the hand.

CLASSICAL INDICATIONS
Back pain, pneumonia, cold and flu, cough, asthma, fibroids, chest pain, fever, palpitations, knee pain, and neck pain.

CLINICAL APPLICATIONS
This point is usually combined with 22.01, however I do not use them often in clinic.

They work best for upper neck pain, especially when there is a blue vein located on the point. It is unclear if the blood congestion makes the points more effective, or if stagnation is showing up in that area. Points 22.01 and 22.02 are a great Dao Ma for upper neck pain, uterine fibroids, and lung issues.

22.02
Chong Xian
Double Saint

These points are typically considered for pain in the area of GB 21. However, I find the results for this to be very random. I do not use them for pain in that area. Point 77.26 is a much better point for this, and it is indicated for pain in the area of GB 21. Points 22.01 and 22.02 should be restricted to pain in the area of C1-7, that is located on the BL channel.

There are many internal indications for these points, they are typically my first choice for pneumonia, bronchial and respiratory issues, and or fevers.

My personal suggestion is to needle Ling Gu deeply, all the way to 22.02. Fan Hou Jue should be needled deeply, all the way to 22.01. Inserting these points in this way is less painful for the patient, and you are also accessing Ling Gu and Fan Hou Jue, which both treat the same indications, and thus would be supporting points. This may not be the traditional way to needle 22.01, 22.02, or Ling Gu and Fan Hou Jue, but to treat upper neck and back pain, lung problems, and lower Jiao stagnation, you will find better clinical results by needling from the dorsal points down into 22.01 and 22.02.

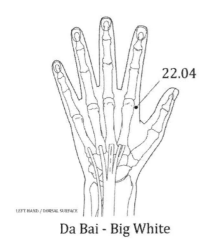

Da Bai - Big White

22.04
Da Bai
Big White

TCM FUNCTIONS
Tonifies the lungs, clears damp phlegm from the lungs, moves Qi and blood, opens the channels and collaterals in the head.

REACTION AREA
Lung

LOCATION AND NEEDLE TECHNIQUE
On the dorsum of the hand, the point is located in the depression 0.5 cun from the joint of the index finger and thumb, or between the first and second metacarpal bones. Lock the fingers in a grip to locate the point. Perpendicular insertion into LI 3.

CLASSICAL INDICATIONS
Childhood asthma, high fever (very effective) and sciatica due to lung deficiency.

CLINICAL APPLICATIONS
This point is one of the most commonly used points in the Tung system. It is used in combination with Ling Gu to create a Dao Ma. A whole book could be written about the clinical application of Ling Gu and Da Bai. Da Bai is used 95% of the time in combination with Ling Gu. The most common uses for Da Bai, when used alone, are headaches and other head problems.

The name Da Bai means big white. The assumption would be that it treats problems such as extreme lung problems, asthma, and respiratory conditions.

22.04
Da Bai
Big White

I don't like to say that any point is effective, regardless of which channel is affected, but Da Bai really is effective to treat headaches on any channel. It treats any headache. That is not good to say, we must always treat the root cause, not the symptom, but Da Bai is that good at treating headaches, so I feel it is safe to say it treats any headache.

The indications for this point include high fever, acute pneumonia, and childhood asthma. You will rarely treat this in your clinic, and if you did, there are better point choices, and herbs are a better option. Clinically Da Bai is better when used in combination with Ling Gu.

I would urge you not to get into the habit of using Da Bai alone, it is best to combine it with Ling Gu. Ling Gu is the primary point, and Da Bai is the assistant point.

Finally, regarding the location of Da Bai. I think the two biggest arguments in the world are "does climate change exist," and "is LI 3 in the same location as Da Bai?"

I would suggest that Da Bai is in the same location as LI 3. That is how Dr. Wei Chieh Young teaches it. If you prefer to find a different location, such as "just proximal to LI 3, under the tendon, before the bone," then use that location.

Use whatever location you were taught for 10-20,000 treatments. Then ask yourself if the point has performed well for you. Has it served your patients? Has it fulfilled your expectations? If it has, keep your location. If it has not, then shift. The definition of insanity is doing the same thing over and over again and expecting a different result.

The location of this point is certainly a big issue with people in Tung acupuncture. One prominent Tung scholar locates 33.13, 33.14, and 33.15 not only in a different location, but on a different channel! According to one notable Tung teacher, it is on the PC channel. I was taught that 33.13, 33.14, and 33.15 are on the LU channel. This is what is ironic, those points on the PC channel have been working for years and years before that particular Tung teacher made his assertions. They have been working on patients, and getting great results!

22.04
Da Bai
Big White

What does this mean to you? It means to follow your teacher, ask questions, and if a point does not work for you after 10,000 treatments at a minimum, you can make a decision for yourself. Ask yourself if it is working for you, and if it is the correct location. What would Master Tung say? Master Tung would tell you to observe and think for yourself.

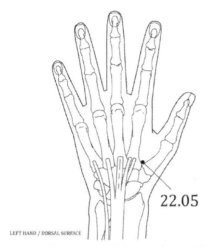

22.05
Ling Gu
Miraculous Bone

(also known as Spirit Bone)

Ling Gu - Miraculous Bone

TCM FUNCTIONS
The indications of this point are endless. As the name of this point suggests, "miracle bone," it is somewhat of a miracle point. It invigorates all five Zang organs, moves Qi and blood, and clears the channels. It expels wind, raises Yang Qi, supports the Yin, and secures the essence. It breaks stagnation and treats phlegm. It is really miraculous.

REACTION AREA
Lung

LOCATION AND NEEDLE TECHNIQUE
The point is located in the junction between the index finger and thumb, the 1st and 2nd metacarpal bones, 1.2 cun from Da Bai (22.04), and directly opposite Chong Xian (22.02). Lock the fingers in a grip to locate the point. The classical way to needle this point is to insert it into the point so the tip of the needle hits the bone of the index finger, the metacarpal bone.

I would suggest there are two other ways to insert this point. You can needle it so it goes under the index finger, and ends up around Yao Tong Xue point, which is a TCM extra point. Basically you needle Ling Gu in the direction of SI 4. In my experience, this is the most effective way to needle this point.

The other way you can needle Ling Gu is to insert the needle in the direction of 22.02. In this way, you will activate both points, Ling Gu and 22.02. I might use this needling method depending on the condition I am treating.

22.05
Ling Gu
Miraculous Bone

CLASSICAL INDICATIONS
Sciatica due to hypofunction of the lungs, lower back pain, foot pain, facial paralysis, hemiplegia, enlargement of bones, irregular menstruation, amenorrhea, difficult labor, back pain, tinnitus, migraine, dysmenorrhea, intestinal pain, dizziness, and a distending sensation of the head.

CLINICAL APPLICATIONS
Ling Gu is the most important point in the Tung system. When in doubt, use Ling Gu. If you don't know what to do, use Ling Gu. There are over 50 indications for Ling Gu, but the most common uses are:

- Raise the Yang Qi, fatigue, blood flow, systemic pain, and systemic blood circulation.
- Hemiplegia
- Any blood flow issue to the head, dizziness, Meniere's, vertigo.
- Bell's palsy
- Headache
- Sciatica, the L5/S1 area, and the ischium area. (Not just lower back pain)
- Shoulder pain
- Elbow pain
- Wrist pain
- Eye issues, such as a sty, and vision problems.
- Hernia, groin, genital, and uterus issues.
- Moves Qi and blood everywhere, in particular in the channels/collaterals, and the head.

Ling Gu treats the bone and KD, so it treats urinary problems
Ling Gu treats the LU, so it tonifies the Qi
Ling Gu treats the LV, so it treats all gynecological issues
Ling Gu treats the KD, so it treats ear issues

Ling Gu plus 88.25 treats any pain of any unknown origin or pathology.

Sciatica

Ling Gu plus GB 41 treats sciatica on the GB channel
Ling Gu plus BL 65 treats sciatica on the BL channel
Ling Gu plus ST 42 treats sciatica on the ST channel

22.05
Ling Gu
Miraculous Bone

There are many more indications for Ling Gu. However, you will see it used most often for:

- Lower back pain
- Blood circulation
- Fatigue
- Headaches
- Reproductive issues
- Diseases of unknown origin, or if the practitioner is confused as to where to start

In my experience, of the 100 people I see each week, I have only one or two who are sensitive to having Ling Gu treated. It is not a painful point.

In conclusion, it is almost a disservice to discuss in a book what Ling Gu is, or what it does. It is that amazing. It is not appropriate to write about it. It has to be felt and experienced. This point is what changed the direction of my acupuncture career. The insertion of this point is the only thing that resolved my chronic back pain.

Of course, we need to write about and discuss this point, but its actions cannot be explained. You need to use it in your practice, on thousands of people to truly understand the magnificence and depth of this point. After 60,000 treatments, I still continue to be astounded by the effect it has on my patients. Writing can only scratch the surface of the power of this point.

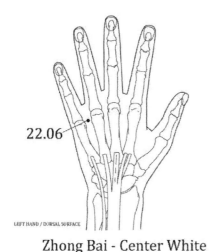

Zhong Bai - Center White

22.06
Zhong Bai
Center White

TCM FUNCTIONS
Tonifies the kidneys, soothes and clears the heart, drains dampness, and tonifies the spleen. Moves Qi and blood, and opens the channels and collaterals, and stops pain.

REACTION AREA
Kidney, Heart, Spleen

LOCATION AND NEEDLE TECHNIQUE
The point is located between the dorsal metacarpal bones of the little and ring fingers, 0.5 cun proximal to the metacarpophalangeal joint. Lock the fingers in a grip to locate the point. Perpendicular insertion.

CLASSICAL INDICATIONS
Lower back ache due to renal problems, back pain, dizziness, astigmatism, fatigue, sciatica due to renal problems, pain on the lateral malleolus, and edema of the limbs.

CLINICAL APPLICATIONS
Combine 22.06 with 22.07. Please refer to 22.07 for clinical applications. Some acupuncturists say that this point is very effective when used alone, which it can be. It is an amazing point. However, for better results, combining these two points is imperative.

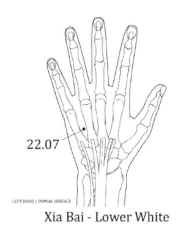

22.07
Xia Bai
Lower White

Xia Bai - Lower White

TCM FUNCTIONS
Tonifies the kidneys, soothes and clears the heart, removes dampness and tonifies the spleen. Moves Qi and blood, opens the channels and collaterals to stop pain.

REACTION AREA
Kidney, Heart, Spleen

LOCATION AND NEEDLE TECHNIQUE
The point is located between the dorsal 4th and 5th metacarpal bones, 1.5 cun proximal to the metacarpophalangeal joint, 1 cun posterior to 22.06 on the dorsal side. Lock the fingers in a grip to locate the point. Insert the needle 0.3-0.5 cun deep. Perpendicular insertion.

CLASSICAL INDICATIONS
Toothache, slight liver pain. This point has the same indications as 22.06. Eye problems, lower back pain, tinnitus, dizziness, edema of the limbs, hypertension, heart palpitations, pain upon sitting or standing, pain in the chest that goes through to the back, blurry vision, fatigue, and headaches.

CLINICAL APPLICATIONS
Points 22.06 and 22.07 are used together. They are some of the most effective points to treat any kidney issue. The TW treats the KD. They also treat the lower back, shoulders, and neck. They are more effective if the pain is located on the TW or GB channels in the upper back and neck.

It is interesting that these points are indicated for pain when bending or sitting, as in pain where your back bends. With kidney pain, kidney stones, or kidney inflammation, it usually hurts very badly when you bend, stand, or sit.

22.07
Xia Bai
Lower White

Your body bends at the L5/S1 joint. To treat that area, Ling Gu is the preferred point. You also bend over at the area of T10. Your kidneys are located in that area. Since these points are on the TW channel, (the TW treats the KD organ and channel), it is very beneficial for patients who have back pain caused by kidney problems, which usually affects the area of T8-12.

Since this point overlaps TW 3 and TW 4, the Shu Stream point, they are the Shao Yang, so they treat the gall bladder. The TW treats the PC (which controls the heart function, which explains the palpitations and tight chest). This is why 22.06 and 22.07 stop pain in the chest that radiates to the back. That's pain from the heart radiating into the upper back. The TW fixes the PC. The PC is the function of the heart.

The TW and KD control water, edema, and the mesenteric artery system, which are all responsible for dampness. The TW interacts with the SP. The TW interacts with the KD. This explains the numerous weak kidney Qi indications, such as dizziness, edema, hypertension, back pain, toothache, eye issues, fatigue, and tinnitus.

The name of this point has "Bai" in it. Bai means white, and white is associated with the lungs. It is interesting to note, because the early stages of hearing loss are considered to be a lung Qi deficiency problem in TCM. The name has white, implying it treats the lungs, which helps hearing. I find this intriguing.

Since we are trying to treat the KD and GB, and the TW treats both of these, and both are connected to the bones, we need to insert our needle close to the bone on these points. Since we know the TW interacts with both the KD and GB, it is also very effective to treat kidney stones or gallstones.

This is a very popular point to treat sciatica, but not just any type of sciatica. It is most effective when the sciatica is on the GB channel. The TW treats the GB. Think of this point as clearing pain along the TW and GB channels.

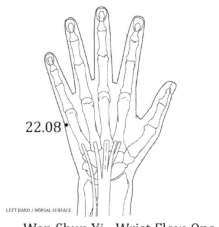

Wan Shun Yi - Wrist Flow, One

22.08
Wan Shun Yi
Wrist Flow, One

TCM FUNCTIONS
Tonifies and invigorates the kidneys. Dispels BL channel pathogens, dispels damp, and clears small intestine damp heat.

REACTION AREA
Kidney

LOCATION AND NEEDLE TECHNIQUE
This point is located on the lateral side of the dorsal 5th metacarpal bone, 2.5 cun distal to the wrist crease. Another way to locate these points is that 22.08 is .5 cun from SI 3, and 22.09 is .5 cun distal to SI 4. Perpendicular insertion

CLASSICAL INDICATIONS
Headache, blurred vision, sciatica due to kidney deficiency, nephritis, edema of the limbs, heaviness and pain on both sides of the lower back, and back pain. This point is especially effective on females, but needle one side only.

CLINICAL APPLICATIONS
This point is always combined with 22.09. Please refer to 22.09 for clinical indications. Point 22.08 is similar to SI 3, whereas 22.09 is similar to SI 4. However, they are very different points with special attributes, beyond just the indications of SI 3 and SI 4.

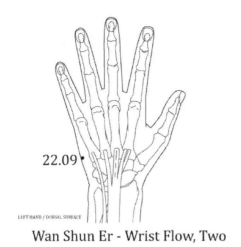

22.09
Wan Shun Er
Wrist Flow, Two

Wan Shun Er - Wrist Flow, Two

TCM FUNCTIONS
Tonifies and invigorates the kidneys. Dispels BL channel pathogens, dispels damp, and clears small intestine damp heat. Tonifies and invigorates the kidneys. Clears BL channel pathogens, dispels damp, and clears small intestine damp heat.

LOCATION AND NEEDLE TECHNIQUE
This point is located on the dorsal side of the lateral side of the 5th metacarpal bone, 1.5 cun distal to the wrist crease. It is 1 cun posterior to 22.08. Insert the needle 1-1.5 cun deep. Perpendicular insertion.

REACTION AREA
Kidney

CLASSICAL INDICATIONS
Nosebleeds, and illness treated by 22.08. Treats headaches, blurred vision, and fatigue, sciatica due to kidney deficiency, edema, nephritis, swollen joints, lower back pain, spinal pain, and pain behind the knee, eye tics, trigeminal neuralgia, and sciatica on the BL channel, toothaches, eye pain, tinnitus, and lower abdominal distension.

CLINICAL APPLICATIONS
Points 22.08 and 22.09 are always used together for better results. They are also very effective for kidney issues, because the SI drains damp, and the relationship of the SI to the KD. The reaction area of these points is the KD. These points are very close to SI 3 and SI 4 and thus have many similar indications as SI 3 and SI 4.

22.09
Wan Shun Er
Wrist Flow, Two

These points are used often for neck and back pain, especially pain that is on the SI, BL, and TW channels. They are very effective for Tai Yang sciatica, and are interestingly wonderful for pain behind the knee cap. They are very effective for back pain on the erector spinae, and the paraspinal muscles of the lower back. They also treat teeth pain and eye problems. Clinically they are not useful for tinnitus.

Due to the indications of tonifying the kidneys and draining damp, they treat fatigue, and swollen, damp, and painful joints. I remember at one seminar Dr. Tan used these points for my back pain on the erector and paraspinal muscles, around the area of L2-5, my pain was instantly gone. Dr. Tan even looked at me and said it was ok if I still hurt he wasn't finished treating my back, but it was instantly better.

Because the fifth finger in Tung acupuncture is associated with the kidneys, and these points cover the reaction area of the kidney, they are wonderful for any kidney related pathology.

As a Dao Ma, 22.08 and 22.09 are especially effective to treat sacral pain.

These points can be used to show how they can treat neck pain and back pain. If you insert a needle in SI 3, which is the TCM master point of the neck, the pain will still persist. If you add 22.08 and 22.09, the lower back pain goes away, and the neck pain is improved.

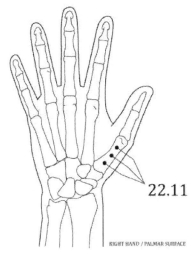

Tu Shui - Earth Water

22.11
Tu Shui
Earth Water

Palmar side

TCM FUNCTIONS
UPPER JIAO
Regulates the Lungs, disinhibits the throat, and reduces fever.

MIDDLE JIAO
Dispels cold and damp from the middle Jiao, warms the center, harmonizes the spleen and stomach, raises sinking stomach Qi.

REACTION AREA
Kidney, Spleen

LOCATION AND NEEDLE TECHNIQUE
On the palmar side of the first metacarpal bone, on the radial side. Roll the needle off the thumb into the crease between the thenar eminence and the thumb bone. These points are tighter to the bone than the traditional location of LU 10. I press for one second on the point, to disperse the blood from the point, as I release, I insert the needle. The needle is inserted at the same angle as LU 10. Insert the needle close along the metacarpal bone.

CLASSICAL INDICATIONS
Gastritis, chronic gastropathy, and gastric ulcer.

22.11
Tu Shui
Earth Water

CLINICAL APPLICATIONS

It is interesting to note that in the Yellow Emperor's Classic it says that the Lung runs to the middle Jiao, travels to the large intestine, and encircles the stomach. This explains why this point is so effective for gastrointestinal diseases.

Even the Ling Shu says the thenar eminence, where these points are located, is used to diagnose stomach conditions. It is commonly referred to as the fish belly. Even Dr. Jimmy Chang, who teaches Chinese herbs and pulse diagnosis, will examine the area of LU 10 and 22.11, to diagnose digestive, upper neck, or back issues.

I even use this point for the common cold, because it is close to LU 10, which is the Ying Spring point on the LU channel. The Ying Spring treats external and channel issues. That is why it is so effective to treat the common cold or other wind issues.

I use these points every day to treat patients with poor digestion that is related to the liver invading the Spleen and Stomach. Common manifestations are diarrhea, upset stomach, loose stools, and dampness in the middle burner, irritable bowel syndrome, Crohn's disease, colitis, and many other types of digestive issues.

Other indications are chronic gastritis, and gastric ulcer. I use these as some of the main points for patients who have loose stools due to removal of their gall bladders.

This is not a top Tung point in the classical sense. However, since so many modern patients have stomach issues, have their gall bladders removed, have loose stools, gas, bloating, or abdominal discomfort, I use these points quite often.

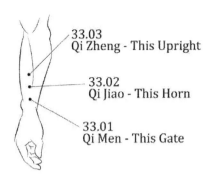

33.03
Qi Zheng - This Upright

33.02
Qi Jiao - This Horn

33.01
Qi Men - This Gate

33.01
Qi Men
This Gate

33.02
Qi Jiao
This Horn

33.03
Qi Zheng
This Upright

Three Qi Dao Ma

TCM FUNCTIONS
Harmonizes the Spleen and Stomach, moves Qi and blood in the middle and lower Jiao, and lifts descending Qi.

REACTION AREA FOR ALL THREE POINTS
Lung

LOCATION AND NEEDLE TECHNIQUE
This point is located on the radial side of the forearm, on the line between LI 5 and LI 11. Point 33.01 is located two cun from the wrist crease. Point 33.02 is two cun proximal to 33.01, 33.03 is two cun proximal to 33.02. Pinch the skin to insert, horizontal insertion, the shaft of the needle should run along the bone. Use a 1.5 inch needle with 1.25 inches inserted. Direct the needle in the direction of LI 11, parallel to the bone.

CLASSICAL INDICATIONS
Irregular menstruation, leukorrhea with reddish discharge, prolapsed rectum, and hemorrhoid pain.

CLINICAL APPLICATION
Points 33.01, 33.02, and 33.03 are always used together. They are used most commonly for gynecological disorders and hemorrhoids. This is explained in part by the relationship between the LI and LV. It is interesting to note that these points are close to the TCM extra point Er Bai, which is considered to be empirically good for hemorrhoids in TCM theory. These points are used primarily for irregular menstruation, since the LI is full of Qi and blood. They are effective for any menstrual disorder.

53

33.01, 33.02 and 33.03

These points have a lifting effect. They lift the distended intestines to treat hemorrhoids. I have used these points to save the life of an unborn baby that was supposed to be born prematurely. These points were crucial in lifting the uterus and child. After childbirth, they can be used to lift the uterus back into its original position.

These points are excellent to treat chronic IBS, spleen and stomach disharmonies, chronic constipation, sluggish bowels, and any stagnation in the groin area, or lower Jiao.

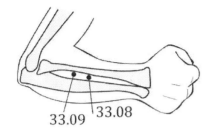

**33.08
Shou Wu Jin
Arm Five Metal**

**33.09
Shou Qian Jin
Arm 1000 Metal**

Two Metal Dao Ma

TCM FUNCTIONS
UPPER JIAO
Tonify Lung Qi.

MIDDLE JIAO
Harmonizes the spleen and stomach, rectifies stomach Qi, regulates liver Qi, and tonifies liver blood.

SYSTEMIC
Treats wind, releases the exterior, moves Qi and blood, stops pain, courses the channels and collaterals.

REACTION AREA
33.08 Lung
33.09 Liver

LOCATION AND NEEDLE TECHNIQUE
Perpendicular insertion 5 fen lateral to the TW channel, on the lateral side of the ulna.
Point 33.08 is 6.5 cun proximal from the wrist crease
Point 33.09 is 8.0 cun proximal from the wrist crease
Point 33.09 is also measured as 1.5 cun proximal to 33.08.

CLASSICAL INDICATIONS
Sciatica, abdominal pain, distending feeling of the leg, and pain and numbness of the feet.

33.08 and 33.09

CLINICAL APPLICATIONS

These points are often underutilized and underappreciated. Points 33.08 and 33.09 are always used together.

They are very effective to treat:

- BL or GB channel sciatica
- Chest pain
- Chest constriction
- Heart issues, and just about any condition on the torso.
- Neuropathy
- Numbness or tingling anywhere in the body.
- Raynaud's
- Rib pain – extremely effective for this
- Systemic blood flow, stagnation, blood issues
- Digestion problem, gas and bloating
- Early stage skin diseases
- External wind diseases
- Wounds
- Skin rash

I will frequently default to these two points if I don't know what to do or where to start, they are good at rebalancing the body. Since most pain is Qi and blood stagnation, I usually use these points to supplement or reinforce my overall treatment plan.

These points are often undervalued clinically. They are extremely effective and are always used together. Since 33.08 and 33.09 are both on the tendon (LV), and the bone (KD), they both treat these organs. Because these points are located between the SI and TW channels, they treat both the SI and TW. These points have many indications and are clinically useful for most patients. Point 33.08 is not used alone.

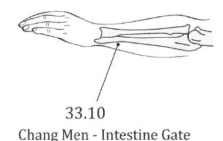

33.10
Chang Men - Intestine Gate

33.10
Chang Men
Intestine Gate

Three Gates Dao
Ma, 33.10-11-12

TCM FUNCTIONS
Regulates and tonifies spleen and stomach Qi, transforms cold damp, and damp heat stagnation in the intestines. Moves and supplements spleen and stomach Qi, transforms cold damp, damp heat, and stagnation in the intestines.

REACTION AREA
Liver, Kidney

LOCATION AND NEEDLE TECHNIQUE
Located on the medial side of the ulna on the SI channel, three cun proximal to the pisiform bone. Insert the needle 0.3-0.5 cun deep. The insertion is perpendicular, since it is on the SI channel, this point can be used as an acupressure point to stop urgent diarrhea.

CLASSICAL INDICATIONS
Enteritis caused by hepatitis, dizziness, blurred vision, abdominal pain, diarrhea, sudden urge to defecate. It stops gas and bloating.

CLINICAL APPLICATIONS
This is a very popular point in the Tung system. Points 33.10, 33.11, and 33.12 are a great three point Dao Ma. These points are usually used together. However, 33.10 is good enough to be used separately.

This point is called Intestine Gate. It will treat all intestinal issues. It is more effective to treat urgent bowel movements than constipation, but it will treat both. I usually combine this with 66.05, as a starting point to treat digestive issues.

This point is also used a lot to treat gallbladder disorders, and poor digestion. It is very effective for digestive issues caused by a gallbladder disorder.

33.10
Chang Men
Intestine Gate

This point is very effective to treat gallbladder related digestive issues that result in poor bile production. This causes intestinal hyper-motility. This point treats weak spleen and stomach, and can also treat damp heat or cold in the middle burner. This can manifest as irritable bowel syndrome, Crohn's disease, gastritis, colitis, diarrhea, constipation, lack of gallbladder causing digestive issues, pancreatitis, fatty liver, sluggish bowels, pain anywhere in the middle or lower Jiao, and feelings of fullness. These are common presentations in Western clinics.

Three Gates Dao Ma

33.10, 33.11, and 33.12

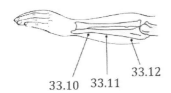

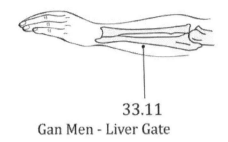

33.11
Gan Men - Liver Gate

33.11
Gan Men
Liver Gate

TCM FUNCTIONS
Regulates Liver Qi and blood, drains damp heat, course the liver and rectifies Qi, quickens the blood and transforms stasis, and stops pain.

REACTION AREA
Liver

LOCATION AND NEEDLE TECHNIQUE
On the ulnar side on the SI channel, 6 cun proximal to the pisiform bone. Perpendicular insertion.

CLASSICAL INDICATIONS
Acute hepatitis

CLINICAL APPLICATIONS
The LV is the most underrated and undertreated organ. With over 600 functions, it is almost as important as the heart. The heart is the emperor organ, but if there were a runner up, it would be the liver.

This point treats the liver. It is also valuable to treat shingles, rib pain, liver issues, fatty liver, and all types of liver organ issues. It is extremely important clinically to treat all liver indications such as fatigue, poor blood flow, and pain in the muscles, tendons, and fascia. Since the liver is on the right side of the body, treating this point on the left side is most effective. It is on the SI channel, and the SI treats the LV.

Since this is on the SI channel, it is close to SI 4, the Yuan Source point, and the SI, it removes turbid damp. It treats the LV, and I expand that clinically to include the definition of the GB. This point treats the LV and GB very effectively.

33.11
Gan Men
Liver Gate

This point is also often effective to treat allergies, infertility, pain, digestion, headaches, fatigue, stress, sleep, neuropathy, edema, hypertension, toxicity, blood flow and hormone issues. In my experience, these issues all originate in a congested and malfunctioning liver. The liver is so compromised that it is affecting the other organs and breaking down a healthy body.

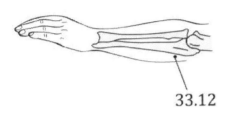

33.12
Xin Men
Heart Gate

33.12

Xin Men - Heart Gate

TCM FUNCTIONS
Regulates heart Qi, removes obstructions, tonifies heart Qi, clears the pericardium, moves Qi and blood, and stops pain. It dispels SI channel pathogens.

REACTION AREA
Heart

LOCATION AND NEEDLE TECHNIQUE
Located in the depression on the medial side of the inferior ulna, 1.5 cun distal to the elbow. It is contraindicated to needle this point bilaterally. Perpendicular insertion. This point is on the SI channel.

CLASSICAL INDICATIONS
Carditis, palpitations, suffocating feeling in the chest, vomiting, and dry cholera. Liver fire rising, knee pain, coccyx pain, groin pain, medial thigh pain, sciatica, and sacral pain.

CLINICAL APPLICATIONS
This is a great point to treat the heart, thus the name, Heart Gate. The SI treats the HT, which is the channel where this point is located. It is used a lot to treat lower back pain, knee pain, coccyx pain, and heart issues.

I often image 33.10 as the lower Jiao, 33.11 as the middle Jiao, and 33.12 as the upper Jiao. This is why these three points are used together to treat many internal disorders in the torso. There are indications of dry cholera, but this condition is not seen in modern clinics. The most common and effective uses of this point are to treat knee pain, coccyx pain, sciatica, lower back pain, groin issues, and heart and chest issues. All these uses are due to the images and channel relationships.

33.12
Xin Men
Heart Gate

This is one of the most commonly used points to treat heart, chest, stress, hypertension, tightness, and pain in the upper chest cavity. Stress and chest tightness sensations are very common in modern clinics. This point can be combined with PC 6, and HT 7 for an effective treatment.

The Dao Ma combination of 33.10, 33.11, and 33.12 is used quite often due to the fact that most patients are affected by poor digestion, liver congestion, and weak hearts. A large proportion of modern patients have issues with these three organs. I have never been disappointed when treating internal disorders with these points.

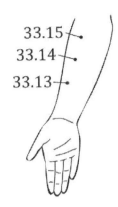

33.15
33.14
33.13

33.13
Ren Shi
Humanity Scholar

33.14
Di Shi
Earth Scholar

33.15
Tian Shi
Heavenly Scholar

Three Scholars Dao Ma

TCM FUNCTIONS

LUNG
Diffuses the lung, dispels cold, courses the channels and frees the connecting vessels. Regulates and tonifies lung Qi. Clears the upper burner.

HEART
Regulates heart Qi, clears the pericardium, clears the upper burner, tonifies heart Qi, quickens the vessels, and frees the channels.

REACTION AREA
Heart, Lung

LOCATION AND NEEDLE TECHNIQUE
Perpendicular insertion.
33.13 is on the LU channel 4 cun proximal from the wrist crease
33.14 is on the LU channel 7 cun proximal from the wrist crease
33.15 in on the LU channel 10 cun proximal from the wrist crease.

CLASSICAL INDICATIONS
Asthma, rhinitis, arm pain, common cold, and suffocating sensation in the chest.

33.13, 33.14, and 33.15

CLINICAL APPLICATIONS

These points are incredible points, and are always used together. They treat all lung issues, allergies, breathing problems, coughing, asthma, a stuffy chest, and any respiratory disease. They are also effective for any heart condition that is caused by a lung dysfunction. I default to these points when I treat any condition related to the lungs.

I often combine 33.13., 33.14, and 33.15 with 1010.19, 1010.20, and 88.17, 88.18, and 88.19. Using three sets of points to treat one issue is a very powerful way to treat any condition. In this case it would be a respiratory or lung Qi disease.

One of the most common reasons patients see a Western medical doctor is to treat breathing problems. Respiratory issues are very common. These points are essential for treating lung problems. These are my first choice to treat coughing.

The LU is wonderful to treat BL problems. The BL channel covers most of the upper and lower back, this is why Master Tung chose the LU channel to treat back pain, like LU 7, LU 9, 22.01 and 22.02.

According to the reaction area, it treats both the heart and the lungs. Master Tung was aware of the special connection that the lung and heart have with each other. The lung grabs the Qi, enriches the Qi, and sends it to the heart to be pumped all over the body. A strong heart cannot exist without strong lungs, and strong lungs cannot exist without a strong heart.

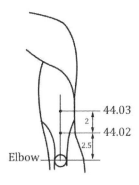

44.02
Hou Zhui
Back Vertebra

44.03
Shou Ying
Head Wisdom

TCM FUNCTIONS
Moves Qi and blood, opens the channels and collaterals, and stops pain. Strengthens the spine. Invigorates and supplements kidney Qi.

REACTION AREA
Liver, Heart, Spine

LOCATION AND NEEDLE TECHNIQUE
Perpendicular insertion. Since we are treating the spine and the kidneys with these points, it is important that the needle touches the posterior side of the humerus.

44.02 – Located on the posterior side of the humerus, 2.5 cun proximal to the cubital crease on the TW channel.

44.03 – Located on the posterior side of the humerus, 4.5 cun proximal to the cubital crease on the TW channel. It is 2 cun proximal from 44.02.

CLASSICAL INDICATIONS
Dislocation, distending pain of the vertebrae, nephritis, hypertension, and lower back pain.

CLINICAL APPLICATIONS
Points 44.02 and 44.03 are not popular Tung points. In my opinion, classically they are not even used as a third or fourth tier points. However, in the modern day clinic, they are extremely important.

44.02 and 44.03

These points are on the TW channel. The TW will treat the KD, which controls the bone and spine. These points also have a reaction area of the spine, Du, Liver and Heart. Most acupuncture visits are for pain, and that pain is usually back pain. The root of that back pain is typically the lower or mid spine. These points are on the mid arm, the mid arm treats the mid back, via the image. The mid arm can also image the lower or upper back, depending on your image.

These points basically treat all issues with the spine, and bulging discs. They are less painful to the patient than the hand points, and clinically I have found they treat a wider range of back problems than 11.11, 11.12, or Ling Gu, for example.

I frequently combine the Bone Spur Points, Gu Ci Yi Er San, with 44.02 and 44.03 to treat mid to lower spine pain, with or without bulging disc issues, degeneration, stenosis, and bone spurs, etc. This is an extremely valuable two point Dao Ma, 44.02 and 44.03, to treat these types of problems.

These points are the top points to treat bulging discs and spine pain. The TW treats the KD. They are clinically exceptional for mid-spine pain in the area of T4-8, and lower back pain in the area of L2-S2. They are also useful for all types of kidney disease, including nephritis.

These points are best known for hypertension and heart issues, polio, and dizziness and headaches from hypertension. I find that acupuncture is great for hypertension, but herbs and lifestyle changes are a necessity. That is why I use these points primarily to treat pain, not heart disease. I do believe that herbs and lifestyle should be the first choice to treat hypertension, while acupuncture plays an important, but secondary role.

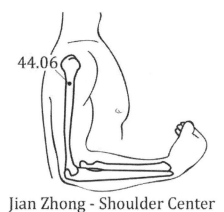

44.06
Jian Zhong
Shoulder Center

Jian Zhong - Shoulder Center

TCM FUNCTIONS
Moves Qi and blood, dispels dampness, tonifies the spleen and stomach, tonifies heart Qi, invigorates the kidneys, releases the exterior, dispels wind in the upper Jiao, stops bleeding, and stops pain.

REACTION AREA
Heart

LOCATION AND NEEDLE TECHNIQUE
On the lateral side of the humerus, 2.5 cun inferior to the acromion joint. Perpendicular insertion. This point is typically found in the middle of medial deltoid in the muscular part.

CLASSICAL INDICATIONS
Knee pain (most effective), dermatosis (most effective for skin diseases in the neck area), polio, hemiplegia, palpitations, arteriosclerosis, nosebleeds, and shoulder pain.

CLINICAL APPLICATIONS
This point is in the top 10-20 points in the Tung system. It is used often for nose conditions, heart conditions, and knee pain. It is also very effective to treat gynecological and fatigue problems. It is valuable for hemiplegia, however there are more effective Tung points to treat this.

Point 44.06 is on the LI channel, and thus influences the LV, the ST (and indirectly the SP), the LU, and the KD. The LI is full of Qi and blood, and this point is located in a big muscle. The muscle is earth, which is the spleen, this explains why it is so effective to treat fatigue and damp disorders.

44.06
Jian Zhong
Shoulder Center

The LI and LV are strongly connected, and thus this point treats so many menstrual disorders. The LV channel encircles the genitals

This is the reaction area of the cardiac nerve, which explains the heart indications. This point is on the LI channel, and the LI treats the ST. Both of the LI and ST have gastro intestinal indications.

I use this point to treat all patients who have fatigue, dampness, spleen and stomach issues, Qi and blood deficiency, or stagnation. I use this point a lot in my practice, at least 10-20 times per day.

Polio is a traditional indication of this point, however I do not remember the last time I saw a case of polio in my American clinic. I have treated polio overseas, but never in America.

When I treat a stuffy nose, fatigue, knee pain, chest and heart problems, which is about 10-20 times a day, 44.06 is always one of my top points. An example of how this point is used is a patient who had right side shoulder pain, in the location of 44.06. I inserted 44.06 on the left side, and then needled GB 31/88.25 on the same side. This is using the theory of treating the pain in the exact location of the pain on the opposite side of the pain. It is not my favorite way to treat, but it is a very fast and easy way to teach someone the most basic way to needle Tung points. Treat the opposite side of the pain, at the exact location of the pain. Always include 88.25 on the same side. It is easy, quick, and usually effective.

Hua Gu Yi - Flower Bone One

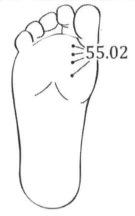

55.02

55.02
Hua Gu Yi
Flower Bone One

Four Flowers Dao Ma

TCM FUNCTIONS
HEAD
Clears wind heat from the eyes and head, brightens and nourishes the eyes. Moves Qi and blood, opens the channels and collaterals in the head, and stops pain.

REACTION AREA
Spleen, Lung, Kidney

LOCATION AND NEEDLE TECHNIQUE
Between the 1st and 2nd metatarsal bones on the plantar surface. If you insert from the traditional location, press on the point firmly, release, and then insert the needle perpendicularly.

An easier, and I think better, way to insert is from the top of the foot at LV 2, LV 2.5, LV 3, and LV 3.5 area through the liver channel down to these points that are on the bottom of the foot. I start from the LV channel and place my non-needle hand under the foot. I insert the needles until I feel the needle tips about to come out on the bottom of the foot. Once I feel that the needle tips are close to the skin surface, which I can feel in my fingers, I stop inserting. The needle is then in the correct location.

CLASSICAL INDICATIONS
Trachoma (Chlamydia trachomatis infection of the eye), ophthalmitis, blepharitis, conjunctivitis, nasal pain, photophobia, tearing on exposure to the wind, headache, toothache, tinnitus, loss of hearing, pain of the nasal bone.

55.02
Hua Gu Yi
Flower Bone One

CLINICAL APPLICATIONS

There is no substitute for these points when it comes to eye issues. I find it best in the clinic to insert from the liver channel through to these points on the bottom of the foot. They are very effective for all head, nose, and eye issues. I usually use only two to three of the four points.

These points are clinically very effective for headaches if you needle down from the LV channel into the area of KD 1. Inserting the needles from the top of the foot in the LV channel activates these points from the top side. The body does not know how you activated the points, they were just activated. Inserting this way activates more channels, covers more indications, and thus has a greater effect.

This theory is why many high level Tung teachers say that they love San Cha San. The reason is that when you insert it deeply, this one point activates San Cha San, plus 22.06, 22.07, TW 2, TW 3, TW 4, SI 3, SI 4, 22.08, and 22.09. Using just one needle, so many points are activated. Inserting the needle down through the LV channel is the same principle.

A great example of how this point can be used is a patient of mine who after only six treatments, has been able to reduce her eyeglass prescription three times. She is now using the glasses prescribed to her from three prescriptions before the most recent one.

Her eyes are improving so much. Her diagnosis is macular degeneration. She had to use some older glasses, because her eyes had improved so much. We joke that every time she shows up she is wearing her old, out of date glasses, because her eyes are getting better and better. She does not need her current glasses. I doubt she will be able to get rid of her glasses entirely. However, her prescription so far has been reduced by 40%.

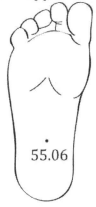

Shang Liu - Upper Tumor

**55.06
Shang Liu
Upper Tumor**

TCM FUNCTIONS

HEAD AND BRAIN AREA
Move Qi and blood, stop pain, drain and dispel damp.

REACTION AREA
Brain

LOCATION AND NEEDLE TECHNIQUE
Located in the center of the anterior edge of the heel. This point is not painful for the patient. Press firmly into the point. Tell your patient it might feel a bit odd, then insert the needle. It is quick and easy, and 99% of the time it is painless. Insertion is perpendicular. I needle young children with brain trauma at this point, and they never complain. It is not that scary.

CLASSICAL INDICATIONS
Brain tumor, headache, swelling of the cerebellum, cranial nerve pain (trigeminal neuralgia), fatigue, stuffy nose, and bleeding from the nose.

CLINICAL APPLICATIONS
This point is very effective for hydrocephalus, brain injury, and trauma. It treats any problem with the head and the brain. This is a microsystem of the head on the foot, where this point is located. A great Dao Ma is KD 1 and 55.06, or KD 2 and 55.06. It is also effective for stuffy nose, bleeding nose, stuffy head, cloudy thinking, heavy head, and brain fog.

55.06
Shang Liu
Upper Tumor

I used this point on a woman with trigeminal neuralgia that resulted from hydrocephalus that was caused by chemotherapy. They inserted a tube in her brain that drained the fluid into her stomach. However, the draining tube they put in her head caused so much pain, that she was in the emergency room 2-3 times per week. Although she had the tube in her head to drain the fluid, she was still dizzy and she now had a headache that she described as an 11 of 10. This point was one of the main points I used to treat this complex issue in four treatments. That is how powerful, simple, easy, fast, and therapeutically effective these Tung points are.

For a patient who had a caffeine withdrawal headache, I was going to use other points, such as 88.12, 88.13, and 88.14, because they treat headaches and the liver. I believed that the liver was the root of her caffeine addiction withdrawal. She said that not only did her head hurt, but it hurt on the inside. She said it felt like her brain was swelling. This to me indicated dampness and swelling in the brain. That led me to use this point. Upon insertion, her headache was gone.

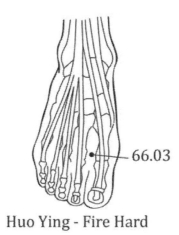

66.03
Huo Ying
Fire Hard

66.03

Huo Ying - Fire Hard

TCM FUNCTIONS
Dispels wind, moves Qi and blood, increases systemic circulation.

UPPER JIAO
Tonifies the heart, moves heart Qi, opens and clears the pericardium.

MIDDLE JIAO
Tonifies the liver, moves liver blood and Qi, and opens the channels and collaterals.

REACTION AREA
Heart, Liver

LOCATION AND NEEDLE TECHNIQUE
Between the 1st and 2nd metatarsal bones, 0.5 cun from the metatarsophalangeal joints, on the dorsal surface. Perpendicular insertion.

CLASSICAL INDICATIONS
Strengthens the heart, an emergency point for fainting or heart attack. Palpitations, tumor of the uterus, uterine fibroids, retained placenta, inflammation of the uterus, chin pain, pain of the temporomandibular joint, grinding teeth from stress, and dizziness.

66.03
Huo Ying
Fire Hard

CLINICAL APPLICATIONS

The name of this point translates as "make the fire harder" and thus we know it improves circulation. To increase the "fire" we are increasing the HT. The LV treats the PC, the PC controls the cardiac function. This point is close to LV 2.

Clinically I use this point all the time to treat TMJ, headaches, circulation issues, heart problems, and any type of bleeding in the groin or gynecological area. Remember that the liver controls the tendons, so the LV should be considered for any tendon issue. The liver also controls the tendon, which includes shaking, and wind. There is also a vessel under this point, the dorsalis pedis artery. Vessel treats vessel, which explains all the circulation, blood flow, Qi and blood stagnation, liver, and heart indications.

This point, combined with 66.04 is very effective for a stuffy nose, not only because of the image and channel, but because of the typical root cause of a stuffy nose. Typically a stuffy nose has no blood flow, it also has phlegm and damp. These points make the fire harder, they drive fire up into the damp, phlegmy, and cold nose, which has no blood circulation, and open it.

This is a secret to Tung points. It can be channel and image, but it is much more than that. It is the channel and image, and also the root, which is the diseased organ. The assumption here is that the root cause of the stuffy nose was improper blood flow, both of which are treated by a stronger heart and liver. It is not enough to know the points treat headaches or stuffy noses, you need to know *why*.

I usually use 66.03 with 66.04. This is a Dao Ma called *Two Fires*. However, 66.03 is a special point and worth mentioning on its own. I strongly suggest that to treat the indications listed for 66.03, you combine it with 66.04. The effect is much better.

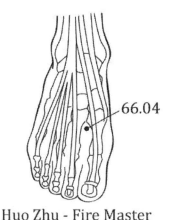
Huo Zhu - Fire Master

66.04
Huo Zhu
Fire Master

TCM FUNCTIONS
Moves Qi and blood, increases systemic circulation, expels wind damp.

UPPER JIAO
Tonifies the heart, moves heart Qi, opens and clears the pericardium, opens the channels and collaterals.

REACTION AREA
Heart

LOCATION AND NEEDLE TECHNIQUE
One cun posterior to 66.03. Perpendicular insertion.   This is as close to the juncture of the 1st and 2nd metatarsal joint as possible.

CLASSICAL INDICATIONS
Emergency point for heart attacks, enlargement of the bones, headache, inflammation or tumors of the uterus, gastrointestinal diseases, liver diseases, neurasthenia, breech presentation, pain in the hands and feet, difficult labor, headache due to heart problems, liver and stomach diseases, inflammation and tumors of the uterus.

66.04
Huo Zhu
Fire Master

CLINICAL APPLICATIONS

In modern clinics, most of our patients have fatigue, stress, tension, Qi and blood stagnation, a congested and weak liver, and either an over-active heart, (hypertension), or an under-active heart (poor circulation). This one point, 66.04, although it is better if combined with 66.03, should be your most commonly used point.

Other indications, that are not Tung, but are amazing nonetheless, is pain in the area of SI 18, SI 17, TW 17, and pain under the eyes, stuffy, congested nose issues, and throat problems. The Classics say the internal branch of the LV channel goes through the throat. Inguinal pain, groin pain, wind damp cold type knee pain.

This point is arguably one of the best points in the Tung system to treat the heart. It is one of the top 10 points of Master Tung, and I use this point almost daily. It is very good for moving Qi and blood, facial pain, headaches, reproductive issues both male and female. Raynaud's, circulatory issues, systemic blood flow issues. I use this point on at least 75% of my patients.

The four gates is what TCM students learn in school to move Qi and blood, relieve stress, and calm the Shen. That treatment is a bilateral LI 4 and LV 3. I would suggest that a more powerful four gates is bilateral Ling Gu (22.05), and bilateral 66.04.

Do not underestimate the importance of any liver point in any system of acupuncture. The liver is one of the most pathological organs in modern culture. It is also one that is frequently overlooked.

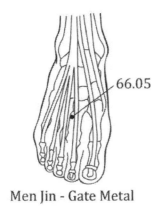

66.05

Men Jin - Gate Metal

66.05
Men Jin
Gate Metal

TCM FUNCTIONS

UPPER JIAO
Clears and soothes Yang Ming channel in the face, harmonizes wood, and the GB channel in the face. Removes obstructions, dispels wind, and drains fire and damp.

MIDDLE JIAO
Strengthens the spleen, disinhibits damp, harmonizes the stomach, and stops rebellious stomach Qi.

LOWER JIAO
Warms the uterus, moves Qi and blood in the lower Jiao, removes obstructions and clears the channels.

REACTION AREA
Stomach, Intestines, Duodenum, Uterus

LOCATION AND NEEDLE TECHNIQUE
This point is at the juncture of the 2nd and 3rd metatarsal bones, the tighter to the junction of the toes you can get the better the point works. Perpendicular insertion.

CLASSICAL INDICATIONS
Enteritis, gastritis, abdominal distension, and appendicitis.

CLINICAL APPLICATIONS
This is a wood point on the earth channel. This explains how it harmonizes so many things, such as the lower Jiao (uterus), the middle Jiao (stomach and intestines), and the upper Jiao (the head, nose, jaw, and eyes).

66.05
Men Jin
Gate Metal

To delve even further into the Five Elements, since this is a wood point, it soothes the liver. That is why we see such wonderful indications for the uterus, painful menstruation, and or headaches, stuffy nose. A congested liver is implicated in all these indications.

This point is very helpful when a patient has a headache, but does not know exactly where it hurts. It is also useful if they feel like their eyeballs are stiff, painful, or they have a headache behind their eyes.

This point is used on most patients with headaches. It is especially useful for pain in the area of Yin Tang, but it is also used for other areas on the head. It is used for any female disorder, or any disorder of the head, TMJ, ear, nose, jaw, etc.

This point is also close to the Shu Stream point, ST 43, and thus has many similar indications and actions such as swelling of the face, edema, rumbling intestines, abdominal pain, persistent cough, night sweating, and redness of the eyes and face. It is definitely one of the Top Ten Tung points.

There are other clinical manifestations that you will commonly encounter that can be treated by this point, depending on the root cause. Migraines (it is especially effective when bled), gastritis, appendicitis, abdominal pain, diarrhea, and dysentery.

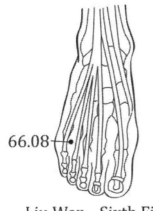

66.08
Liu Wan
Sixth Finish

Liu Wan - Sixth Finish

TCM FUNCTIONS
Clears the liver and gallbladder, brightens the eyes, and sharpens hearing. Clears heat, extinguishes wind and relieves pain. Moves Qi and blood, opens the channels and collaterals.

REACTION AREA
Lung, Kidney

LOCATION AND NEEDLE TECHNIQUE
Between the 4th and 5th metatarsal bones, 0.5 cun proximal to the metatarsophalangeal joint. Perpendicular insertion. Point 66.08 is very close to GB 42.

CLASSICAL INDICATIONS
Hemostasis (including bleeding due to traumatic injury, incised wound, or injection), and migraine headaches.

CLINICAL APPLICATIONS
I always use 66.08 and 66.09 together. These points are used very often in the Tung system. I use them primarily for systemic bone swelling, systemic inflammation, and headaches. These points are great when your patient says her whole body hurts. Point 66.08 is an amazing point, and it can be used alone, but your success rate with any condition for which these points are indicated, will increase tenfold if you combine 66.08 and 66.09. Please see 66.09 for further explanation.

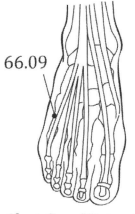

Shui Qu - Water Bend

66.09
Shui Qu
Water Bend

TCM FUNCTIONS
Clears the liver and gall bladder, brightens the eyes, and sharpens hearing.
Clears heat, extinguishes wind, relieves pain, moves Qi and blood, opens the channels and collaterals.

REACTION AREA
Lung, Kidney

LOCATION AND NEEDLE TECHNIQUE
One cun proximal to 66.08. Perpendicular insertion. This point is as tight as you can get to the juncture of the 4th and 5th toes at the proximal metatarsal joint.

CLASSICAL INDICATIONS
Hemostasis (including bleeding due to traumatic injury, incised wound, or injection), and migraine headaches. Lower back pain, peripheral edema, swelling (removes fluid from the body), abdominal distension, generalized joint pain, neck pain, neuralgia of the neck, and uterine disorders.

CLINICAL APPLICATIONS
66.08 has an astringing action and thus is not used on people who have breathing issues, such as asthma. I always use 66.08 and 66.09 together.

66.09
Shui Qu
Water Bend

Points 66.08 and 66.09 are very commonly used in the Tung system. Clinically I use these points most to treat systemic bone swelling, systemic inflammation, and headaches. These points are great when your patient says her whole body hurts.

Although these points are amazing for tinnitus, in my experience your success rate will be below 20% when using acupuncture alone for this. It is very challenging to treat all tinnitus patients. Sometimes you are successful, sometimes you are not. It is not dependable enough.

The theories about these points are rich and deep. Since the needle is close to the bone, we are activating the kidney (water), which treats edema and swelling. The name of the point implies "water cure," hence the treatment of the water/kidney.

It is on a Wood meridian, so the tendons and LV are treated. It is close to a Shu stream point, so the heaviness, swelling, pain, and wind pain which comes and goes. It is on the GB channel, the Shao Yang. The Shao Yang is bone via the Ling Shu, so it treats bone pain all over the body. It is adjacent to the extra meridian, the Dai Mai vessel, so it treats many digestion issues.

GB 41, GB 42, and GB 43 are very popular and powerful points in TCM. In a similar way, 66.08 and 66.09 are just as strong, if not stronger points. This is one of the nuisances of the Tung system. The points are close to GB 41, and it *does* matter if your location is a bit off. It actually does matter. That is where your "good needle becomes a great needle." Rarely in acupuncture is something good or bad. As in my needle is amazing, but your needle is worthless. In most cases, acupuncture still helps the body. However, this is where practitioners go from mediocre to amazing. By changing small things, an "average needle" will become a "miraculous healing needle."

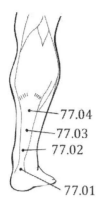

77.01
Zheng Jin
Upright Tendon

77.02
Zheng Zong
Upright Ancestor

77.03
Zheng Shi
Upright Master

77.04
Bo Qiu
Catching Ball

Straight Spine Dao Ma

TCM FUNCTIONS
Moves Qi and blood, stops pain, and opens the Du channel, and spine.

REACTION AREA
Brain, Spine

LOCATION AND NEEDLE TECHNIQUE
In the center of the calcaneus tendon, 3.5 cun superior to the heel. Perpendicular insertion. You must tap the posterior side of the tibia. Insert the needle through the Achilles tendon. It does not matter what position the patient is in, he can be standing, sitting, lying down, face down or face up. The position does not matter. Just ensure the needle is perpendicular, insert through the Achilles tendon, and touch the posterior side of the tibia.

77.01 is 3.5 cun superior to the sole of the foot between the KD and BL, on the Achilles tendon. At the level of the tip of the lateral malleolus and BL 60. Other authors locate this point on a range of 2.5 to 4.5 cun from the sole of the foot.

77.02 is two cun superior to 77.01

77.03 is two cun superior to 77.02

77.04 is two and a half cun superior to 77.03

CLASSICAL INDICATIONS

Neck pain or sprain, spinal pain, neck rigidity, lower back pain, vertebral pain due to sprain, lumbar vertebral pain, neck pain and rigidity and cranial enlargement and hydrocephalus. Pain in the shoulder and back, lower back pain, and sciatica

CLINICAL APPLICATIONS

Points 77.01, 77.02, and 77.03, and 77.04 are always used in combination. I find that using 2 or 3 of the points is sufficient, but sometimes I do use all 4 points if necessary.

These are your first choice to treat neck pain on the bone, cervical issues from C1 to C7, and thoracic from T1 to T4.

In the clinic I typically use the points as follows:
77.01 treats C1-2
77.02 treats C2-4
77.03 treats C4-7/T1
77.04 treats T1-T4

These points clinically treat the spine, the Du and Bladder channels on the neck. I often combine these points with Ren 24 to treat neck pain. (Master Tung was a master at the 14 TCM channels. It is fine to use Tung points with your TCM points. You just need to know the healing mechanisms and when it *is* and is *not* appropriate to combine TCM and Tung points.

These points are effective to treat lower back pain, due to the image and the channel, and for brain problems, due to the reaction area. I love these points for these conditions. They are powerful, effective, and *not* painful. The key to using these points effectively is that you must *tap the bone* on insertion. Needle through the tendon, all the way to the bone. That is key.

Since you insert the needle through the tendon and touch the bone, these points treat the tendon and the bone. The neck is usually stiff due to tendon, muscle or bone problems.

I have yet to see neck pain that originates in the area of C1-T4 on the spine, and BL channels that is not resolved by using these points. These points should be treated on the opposite side. It is best to treat the opposite side, because the points are on the BL channel, and in theory the same channel treats itself on the same side. The BL treats the BL.

77.01 to 77.04

Some people might ask about the Du channel on the spine. This is not the BL treating the Du channel. These points are used regardless of the channel involved. They are so effective that you do not need to consider channel relationships. They treat the spine on the neck, and the upper back. They are simple, effective, and consistent.

When I treated neck pain in India, the pain was usually from trauma, manual labor, or using the head as a tool, such as using it to carry bricks on the top of the head. The people who I did treat for upper back and neck pain in the muscles, were people who had hurt their cervicals or upper thoracic, and the pain was radiating into their GB 21 area.

An example of this was a patient who picked rice all day. He squatted and was constantly looking down, which put pressure on the area of C7/T1. Many other patients carried bricks on their heads while working on construction sites. The women carried their washing on their heads, when walking to and from the rivers to clean. Things like this put pressure on, and damaged the spine, which caused pain that radiated to the muscles. This is an example of treating pain in the area of GB 21 that originated in the spine.

I have noticed that most of the Tung points that are used to treat the upper back and neck, do so by treating the spine. The root of the pain that is treated by 77.01, 77.02, 77.03, 11.11, 11.12, 11.09, Fan Hou Jue, 22.01, 22.02, 22.08, 22.09, 77.05, 77.06, 77.07, are all focused on the spine itself. These points treat the root of the problem, which is the bones.

A recent patient I treated had pain in the area of GB 21. I was not able to help her using other distal points. However, when I inserted 77.01, 77.02, and 77.03, her pain was instantly gone. This was due to the fact that her GB 21 pain was originating from her cervical spine.

I think that Master Tung saw the same type of hard-working, physical labor patients that when they had upper neck and back pain, the root was from the compression, inflammation, and stagnation of the spine. That explains why the points for the upper back, except 77.26, all work because they focus on the spine, which is causing pain to radiate into the upper back muscles.

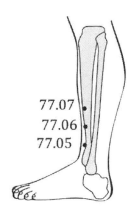

77.05
Yi Zhong
First Weight

77.06
Er Zhong
Second Weight

77.07
San Zhong
Third Weight

Three Weights Dao Ma

TCM FUNCTIONS
This is one of the best points to break and move stuck Qi and blood. It frees the channels and quickens the connecting vessels, stops pain, expels wind, tonifies and clears the spleen. It dispels wind and resolves phlegm.

REACTION AREA
Heart, Lung, Spleen

LOCATION AND NEEDLE TECHNIQUE
Perpendicular insertion between the GB and ST channels. Although the needle is perpendicular, it is really at a 45 degree angle as it goes into the interosseous membrane, between the tibia and fibula.

Located between the ST and GB channels.
77.05 is 3 cun proximal to the lateral malleolus, and 1 cun anterior to the fibula
77.06 is 2 cun proximal to 77.05
77.07 is 2 cun proximal to 77.06

CLASSICAL INDICATIONS
Hyperthyroidism, tonsillitis, deviation of the eye and mouth (facial hemiparesis), migraine headaches, mastitis, fibrocystic breast disease, breast tumors, meningitis, liver disease, splenomegaly, lateral side rib pain, abnormally bulging eyes, lumps, and cranial tumors.

77.05 to 77.07

CLINICAL APPLICATIONS

These will be some of your most frequently used points in clinic, for a few reasons. The first reason is that they are amazing at treating any type of systemic stagnation, blockage, or Qi deficiency. Most of our patients have those as root causes of their diseases. The second reason is that they are very effective to treat neck pain. The type of neck pain they treat is scalene pain, and also to some extent, pain in the area of GB 21.

It is interesting to note that Master Tung told his students to needle these points on the right side. You might ask why. Upon further analysis, the reaction area and nerve of these points is the spleen. The spleen is located on the left side of the body. Although most Tung points are treated on the opposite side, it makes sense that these points were treated on the right side. The original usage of these points was spleen issues. It is very interesting when you break it down into the reasons why this side was chosen.

These points treat wind in the GB channel. They treat phlegm in the ST channel. They are close to GB 39, which treats bone marrow. These Three Weight points treat blood diseases. They regulate the earth and wood, the ST and GB.

These points effectively treat both hyperthyroid and hypothyroid. Not only do the channels go to the neck, but the points image the thyroid correctly. This is in addition to the phlegm, wind, Qi, and blood aspects.

These points are better for scalene issues than for problems in the area of GB 21 and TW 15. Since these points move so much Qi and blood, they are wonderful for many liver issues, and are indicated for cirrhosis, fatty liver, and fatigued liver.

These points have been tested with MRI imaging, and have been verified to increase blood circulation to the head. This explains the indications of hemiplegia, wind stroke, head trauma, headaches, neck pain, and upper back pain.

I use these points all the time to treat migraine headaches, trigeminal neuralgia, tooth pain, tight jaw muscles, TMJ, shoulder pain, and upper back pain, because of their ability to move Qi and blood, dispel wind, and resolve phlegm.

Although this is not a top point in the Tung system, classically it was used primarily to treat spleen problems. However, in our modern clinics, I would suggest that 90 - 95% of your patients will benefit from these points.

A nice example of the usage of this point is a patient who came in with neck pain that was radiating down her arm, into her elbow. This was not classical neck pain. It was pain that only occurred when she breathed in or out. This is interesting, because 77.05, 77.06, and 77.07 treat pain that is associated with the scalene muscles. The scalene muscles are known as the "second breathing muscles." I used 77.01, 77.02, and 77.03 on her with no effect. Upon realizing that her neck pain was caused by the scalene muscles and affected by breathing, I used 77.05, 77.06, and 77.07 and the pain was resolved immediately.

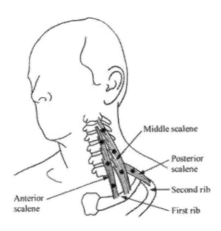

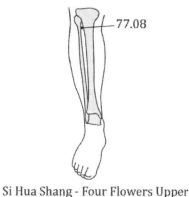
77.08

77.08
Si Hua Shang
Four Flowers Upper

Si Hua Shang - Four Flowers Upper

TCM FUNCTIONS
Dispels wind and phlegm, wind damp, rectifies the spleen and stomach Qi, and regulates central Qi. It supports, corrects, and stores up the original Qi (source Qi), dispels pathogens, and prevents disease. It tonifies lung qi, clears the pericardium, and opens and frees the chest.

REACTION AREA
Lung, Heart

LOCATION AND NEEDLE TECHNIQUE
Three cun inferior to ST 35 on the lateral tibia. The trick to locating this point is to get as close to the tibia as you can. The closer to the bone, the better. This is known as bone shaving, bone cutting, or alleviating bone spurs technique.

Although some texts cite different depths having different functions, this is not my experience. In my experience, you must get the Qi with patients. Since there are so many anatomical differences in our patients, I have found that the clinical references to needle depth and functions do not hold true. You should feel a sensation at the end of your needle, a muscle grab or some other indication that you have the Qi, at any depth of insertion. Although in most cases we have cited the point depths of classical references, getting the Qi is the most important objective.

CLASSICAL INDICATIONS
Asthma, toothache, dizziness, palpitations, coronary artery disease, vomiting, and sudden turmoil.

77.08
Si Hua Shang
Four Flowers Upper

CLINICAL APPLICATIONS

This point is in the top three points in the Tung system. It is very close to ST 36, and it has many of the same indications. The difference for the Tung system is that this point is on the heart line, branch, and reaction area. This is why it is very effective to treat heart and lung issues, Bell's palsy, hemiplegia, jaw problems, teeth issues, face problems, and digestive issues. I use this point on most patients.

Most patients have fatigue. Since this point is an earth point on the earth channel, it is tonifying. The TCM name is Leg Three Mile, which means that we can walk an additional three miles after this point is needled.

It is an amazing point for any face problem, wind attack, headache, tooth or eye problem due to the channel relationships and the images. Since it has the reaction area of the heart and lungs, and the ST channel runs up the leg and chest, it is great for all respiratory diseases. It treats weak lung Qi, and weak heart Qi. It also treats Western defined heart diseases.

This point dispels wind and phlegm, so it will treat many odd diseases. It treats Qi and blood stagnation of any type. Due to the channel and image, it will treat all spleen and stomach disharmonies, and Western gastrointestinal disease. It is an amazing point. It is located closer to the bone than the traditional St 36. Since it is closer to the tibia, the neural network is tighter and denser, which gives it a stronger reflex action on the brain.

This is usually used with 2-3 additional Tung points, like 77.09 and 77.10. However, this point is extraordinary on its own. This point, unlike many others, can stand on its own. Considering how many patients have fatigue, digestion problems, respiratory and emotional issues, and Qi and blood circulation problems, I use it on at least 90% of my patients.

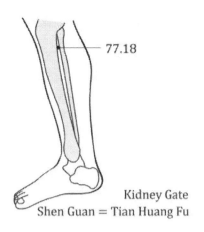

Kidney Gate
Shen Guan = Tian Huang Fu

77.18
Shen Guan
Kidney Gate

also called:
Tian Huang Fu

TCM FUNCTIONS
Supplements the kidneys, dispels wind damp, strengthens the lumbar area and spine, invigorates the heart, and supplements and tonifies the spleen and stomach.

MIDDLE JIAO
Supplements the spleen, resolves Qi stagnation, courses the middle and lower Jiao, dispels wind and damp from the channels and connecting vessels.

LOWER JIAO
Warms and regulates the lower Jiao, dispels cold damp, and eliminates cold in the lower Jiao. It regulates original Qi and prevents disease.

REACTION AREA
Kidney

LOCATION AND NEEDLE TECHNIQUE
Perpendicular insertion, this point is 1.5 cun distal to SP 9. SP 9 in the Tung system is called 77.17. SP 9 (77.17) is often combined with 77.18. To find 77.18 we must find SP 9 first. It just makes sense to needle both together. Insert the needle 1-2 cun deep.

CLASSICAL INDICATIONS
Edema, kidney disease, diabetes mellitus, strangury, premature ejaculation, impotence, seminal emission, nocturnal emission, hematuria, uterine tumors, nephritis, edema of the limbs, proteinuria, irregular menstruation, and lower back pain due to kidney deficiency. Trigeminal neuralgia, fatigue and weakness, general digestive problems, gynecological disorders, and male genital problems such as prostate issues.

77.18
Shen Guan
Kidney Gate

This is the main point for supplementing the kidneys. It treats excess stomach acid, acid reflux, deviation of the eye, astigmatism, dizziness, vertigo, epilepsy, pain in the supraorbital bone, pain in the nasal bone, dark rings under the eyelids, astigmatism, anemia, epilepsy, and neuropathy.

CLINICAL APPLICATIONS
This point is usually combined with 77.19, and 77.21. This forms a Dao Ma called the Three Emperors.

We could write an entire book on Ling Gu and Da Bai, due to the richness of the theory and application of these points. I will try to present a few general theories as to why so many things are treated by these points, but I implore you to always continue your own personal education. You should work through each indication and consider why it works, as I have done.

I often combine 77.18 with SP 9. I rarely use 77.19 alone. If I don't use 77.21 and 77.19 with 77.18, then I will always include SP 9 to create a Dao Ma.

The spleen connects to the kidneys. That is earth connecting to water. You will find that most tonification points in the Tung system are on the SP channel. They support and astringe the KD, to help stop the loss of essence.

The spleen connects with the heart, and thus will treat many sleep and stress disorders. The spleen, 77.18, is close to SP 9, which is the He Sea point, thus these points are used for storing Qi, where Yang Qi enters.

Point 77.21, is close to SP 6, the Three Leg Yin Crossing Point, and it thus affects urogenital disorders. The spleen, earth, is responsible for the middle burner, which is the SP and ST Qi. The three points cover the entire body via the image, which is the full image, half image, and quarter image.

These points treat all issues arising from weak kidneys, as defined by Western medicine and Eastern medicine.

77.18
Shen Guan
Kidney Gate

They are famous for treating frozen shoulder pain. I would suggest they are great for frozen shoulder pain because of the effect they have on cold damp, obstruction of the channels, Qi stagnation, and channel blockages on the LU, SI, and TW channels. It is not just due to the effect on "frozen shoulder."

Dao Ma 77.18, 77.19, and 77.21
You will use these points (77.18-19-21) day in and day out to treat all sorts of back pain, digestive issues, urogenital issues, fatigue, malaise, general aches and pains, general weakness, numbness, cold and damp swelling of the joints, and any type of inflammation, including bursitis, arthritis, and tendonitis.

Points 88.09, 88.10, and 88.11
Many who are familiar with the Tung system will ask why the points 88.09, 88.10, and 88.11 were not included in this book. These points function like 77.18, 77.19, and 77.21. I chose to only include one of the Dao Mas. Since 77.18-19-21 are on the lower leg and easier to access easily, I decided to choose points 77.18-19-21. I find personally in the clinic that even though 77.18, 77.19, 77.21 and 88.09, 88.10, and 88.11 function in a similar way, are on the same channel, have the same indications, actions and same uses, the Three Emperors, 77.18, 77.19, 77.21 are clinically more effective.

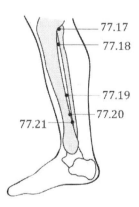

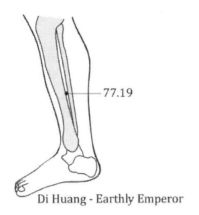

77.19
Di Huang
Earthly Emperor

Di Huang - Earthly Emperor

TCM FUNCTIONS
Supplements the kidney, dispels wind damp, strengthens the lumbar area and spine, boosts the kidneys, invigorates the heart, supplements and tonifies the spleen and stomach.

REACTION AREA
Kidney

LOCATION AND NEEDLE TECHNIQUE
Located 7 cun proximal to the tip of the medial malleolus, on the SP channel. Perpendicular insertion.

CLASSICAL INDICATIONS
Edema, kidney disease, diabetes mellitus, strangury, premature ejaculation, impotence, seminal emission, nocturnal emission, hematuria, uterine tumors, nephritis, edema of the limbs, proteinuria, tumors of the uterus, irregular menstruation, lower back pain due to kidney deficiency.

CLINICAL APPLICATIONS
This point is usually combined with 77.18, and 77.21. Please refer to 77.18 for further information.

This point is very close to SP 7 and it reminds me of something that happened when I observed Dr. Tan in his clinic. One time he had a patient who had tongue pain. In Tung acupuncture we should instantly think that the tongue is muscle, and the muscle is spleen. That would be 1010.22, Bi Yi. It is also the reaction area of the spleen. It's perfect, we have a point that has a tongue indication, and it also fits the root, because the reaction area is the spleen, which is connected to the tongue.

93

77.19
Di Huang
Earthly Emperor

I don't know if Dr. Tan would have used that point or not. On this day in clinic, he did not. He inserted two needles into SP 7, and the woman's tongue pain was instantly gone! I am mentioning this because the relationship of the SP is the clock neighbor of the HT, in system five. I personally hate system five, and I never use it. Here I was, witnessing a wonderful, simple, beautiful, and medically speaking, a fantastic treatment. The patient was 100% happy and thrilled her tongue did not hurt.

This treatment stood out, and I still remember it since that day in 2004. It reminds me to adapt and change. That patient was very apprehensive. I can imagine that I was going to needle her nose, where 1010.22 is located. Regardless of the outcome, I can almost guarantee she would never have returned.

Second, and more importantly, I am constantly reminded to not get so stuck in "theory," or in a way of thinking, no matter what it is. There are many theories, and there are many different opinions on those theories. Sometimes people feel the need for their theory to be superior to another theory, so they staunchly defend it. What really matters? That the point worked! The patient was happy. That is what counts.

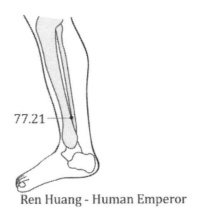

77.21
Ren Huang
Human Emperor

Ren Huang - Human Emperor

TCM FUNCTIONS
Supplements the kidneys, dispels wind damp, strengthens the lumbar and spine, invigorates the heart, and supplements the spleen and stomach.

MIDDLE JIAO
Supplements the spleen, frees Qi stagnation, courses the middle and lower Jiao, and dispels wind damp from the channels and connecting vessels.

LOWER JIAO
Warms and regulates the lower Jiao, dispels cold damp and eliminates cold in the lower Jiao. Regulates original Qi and prevents disease.

REACTION AREA
Kidney

LOCATION AND NEEDLE TECHNIQUE
Located three cun above the tip of the medial malleolus, on the SP channel. Located at SP 6. Perpendicular insertion.

CLASSICAL INDICATIONS
Edema, kidney disease, diabetes mellitus, strangury, premature ejaculation, impotence, seminal emission, nocturnal emission, hematuria, uterine tumors, nephritis, proteinuria, irregular menstruation, and lower back pain due to deficiency of the kidneys. Trigeminal neuralgia, fatigue and weakness, general digestive and gynecological disorders. This point is very close to SP 6, and thus it has many of the same indications of that point.

77.21
Ren Huang
Human Emperor

This point is used more often than 77.19. The point 77.19 functions a bit like SP 7 and 77.21 functions a bit like SP 6. SP 6 is used a lot more than SP 7, so I would suggest that 77.19 is somewhat of an auxiliary point in this Dao Ma. Point 77.18 is the main point, and 77.21 is the supporting point. Point 77.19 facilitates both of these points.

CLINICAL APPLICATIONS

This point is used in combination with 77.18 and 77.19 the majority of the time. Please refer to 77.18 for further information.

I do use this point at times on its own, it functions like SP 6, the 3 leg yin crossing point and is very powerful and effective for SP 6 actions and indications.

I frequently use 77.21 for insomnia, upper back pain, trapezius pain, supraspinatus pain in the upper back, groin, sexual issues in both men and women, reproductive issues in both men and women, stress, and weak kidney or adrenal function.

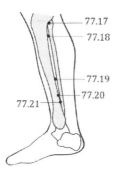

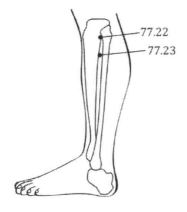

77.22
Ce San Li
Beside Three Miles

77.23
Ce Xia San Li
Distal to Beside Three Miles

TCM FUNCTIONS
Soothes the sinews and vessels, moves and regulates Qi and blood, expels wind from the face, clears damp stagnation in the channels and connecting vessels.

REACTION AREA
Teeth, Lung

LOCATION AND NEEDLE TECHNIQUE
Point 77.22 is 1.5 cun lateral to ST 36. Point 77.23 is 2 cun distal to 77.22, on the anterior border of the fibula. Perpendicular insertion. Both of these points are between the ST and GB channels.

The trick to locating these points is to first find ST 36 using one hand, then find GB 34 with the other hand. Since GB 34 is more proximal than ST 36, move the hand that is touching GB 34 down the GB channel until it is at the same level as ST 36. The first point is located between that GB point and ST 36.

CLASSICAL INDICATIONS
Toothache, facial paralysis, headache, sinusitis, trigeminal neuralgia, Bell's palsy, carpal tunnel, teeth and mouth problems, heel pain, and facial tics.

CLINICAL APPLICATIONS
I always combine 77.22 and 77.23. These are very famous and popular points. I use them all the time for headaches, and because of the reaction area, for the teeth. They are great points for TMJ, and pain in the teeth or mouth.

These should be your first point choice for headaches. Although they are popular for wrist and heel pain, I personally find other points to be better for that.

77.22 and 77.23

These points, since they are located between the Shao yang (GB) which is for wind, shaking, and the bones, and the Yang Ming (ST), which is full of the most Qi and blood, have many clinical uses. There are many unique concepts in the Tung family system of points, and in this case, treating points that lie between channels is similar to blending paint. Our points have attributes of both colors, of both the Yang Ming (ST), and Shao Yang channels (GB).

The reason these points are used so often is that since they treat migraine headaches, headaches in general, TMJ, Qi and blood stagnation, Wind, the LV or GB, and they treat numerous channels that run to the face, which are such common complaints in our clinics. These points are incredibly useful, pain-free to treat, and effective.

These points can be used for heel and wrist pain but they are not my first choice and other points should be chosen.

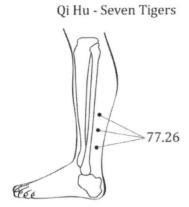

Qi Hu - Seven Tigers

77.26
Qi Hu
Seven Tigers

TCM FUNCTIONS
Regulates Qi and blood, relieves pain, removes obstructions, opens the channels and collaterals, and transforms blood stasis. Opens the chest and sternum, rectifies Qi, regulates the lung, and clears heat.

REACTION AREA
Chest, Thoracic cage

LOCATION AND NEEDLE TECHNIQUE
Located 1.5 cun posterior to the lateral malleolus, on the BL channel. The first point is 2 cun above the tip of the lateral malleolus, the second point is 4 cun above the tip, and the third is 6 cun above the tip. Located behind the posterior border of the fibula.

CLASSICAL INDICATIONS
Sternum pain, clavicle pain, rib pain, and pleurisy.

CLINICAL APPLICATIONS
These are among the few points that are truly indicated to treat pain at GB 21. It is interesting to note that these points are on the BL channel. How can they treat GB 21 pain? Master Tung was aware of the Jing Jin and Tendino-muscular relationships. According to this theory, the trapezius muscles are *not* on the GB channel, but on the BL channel. These Tung points for trapezius pain are on the BL channel.

77.26
Qi Hu
Seven Tigers

Another clinical application is to treat the diaphragm, chest, and breathing issues. The reaction area is the chest. These points are especially effective to treat breathing issues, and chest constriction. They are also indicated for clavicle pain.

For upper back pain, these points should be the first points to consider. The points can be used on either side, but I usually treat them on the same side, since they are on the BL channel, and the BL controls the trapezius area, which is a same side and same channel treatment.

It is interesting to note that chronic pain affects the kidneys. We know that the KD controls the deeper and more chronic muscle problems that are below the more superficial trapezius muscles. The trapezius is the muscle to focus on for more acute and superficial muscle problems. When the pain is chronic, it makes more sense to treat the opposite side, as Master Tung would have suggested. The reason for this is that the KD controls the deeper muscles, which are more affected by chronic issues, which is treated by the BL channel using the Tendinomuscular or Jing Jin channel relationships. The BL treats the KD.

Additional indications are pain in the ribs, lungs, or chest area, scapula pain, and inflammation of the clavicle. This includes such manifestations as pleurisy, chest constriction, painful breathing, and pain at the intercostal muscles.

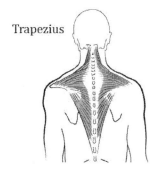

Trapezius

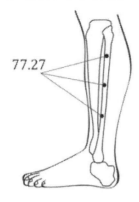

77.27
Wai San Guan
Outer Three Gates

Three Lateral Passes Dao Ma

TCM FUNCTIONS
Dispels all types of wind. This can manifest as heat or cold in the affected tissues. Clears heat, wind, cold, and damp from any trauma. Moves Qi and blood, unblocks the channels and collaterals, stops pain.

REACTION AREA
Lung

LOCATION AND NEEDLE TECHNIQUE
This is a three point unit, located on the line that connects the head of the fibula and the lateral malleolus. The points are located at the ¼, ½, and ¾ units. Perpendicular insertion on the tibia, on the gallbladder channel. The needles must tap the tibia for the best results. Insert the needle 1 to 1.5 cun deep.

CLASSICAL INDICATIONS
Tonsillitis, mumps, laryngitis, abscesses, tumors, and pain in the shoulder and arm.

CLINICAL APPLICATIONS
These points are very strong. They are similar to 77.05, 77.06, and 77.07, in that they treat all systemic stagnation, Qi stagnation, blockages, masses, tumors, injuries from trauma. I often alternate between 77.27 and 77.05, 77.06, and 77.07.

Point 77.27 can be used for any type of trauma, pain, or injury, regardless of the location. They are very effective to treat any type of systemic pain, blockage, or trauma.

77.27
Wai San Guan
Outer Three Gates

I use these points a lot for shingles, rib pain, chest pain, and GB or LV issues. There are many occasions to use these points, depending on the root of the pathology and how the symptoms manifest.

Some common indications are: tonsillitis, tumor, cancer, pharyngitis, and pain in the shoulder or arm. Mumps, laryngitis, abscesses, tumors, fibrocystic breasts, acne, trigeminal neuralgia, swollen hands and arms, and elbow pain.

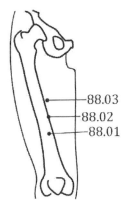

88.01
Tong Guan
Penetrating Gate

88.02
Tong Shan
Penetrating Mountain

88.03
Tong Tian
Penetrating Heaven

Three Penetrations Dao Ma

TCM FUNCTIONS
Points 88.01, 88.02, and 88.03 are always used together.

UPPER JIAO
Rectifies Qi, loosens the chest, regulates Qi and blood, clears the channels and removes obstructions. Regulates heart Qi, clears the pericardium, nourishes the heart, clears heart fire, opens cardiac portals, moves damp, clears edema. It is used for general blood deficiency patterns.

MIDDLE JIAO
Regulates the spleen and stomach, harmonizes the middle Jiao, rectifies central Qi, harmonizes the spleen and stomach, and disperses stagnation

REACTION AREA
Heart

LOCATION and NEEDLE TECHNIQUE
88.01 is located on the anterior midline of the femur, 5 cun superior to the knee crease.
88.02 is located 2 cun more proximal, or a total of 7 cun proximal from the knee crease.
88.03 is located 2 cun more proximal or a total of 9 cun proximal from the knee crease.
Perpendicular insertion.

88.01, 88.02, and 88.03

CLASSICAL INDICATIONS
Heart disease, pericardial pain, pain on both sides of the heart, dizziness, vertigo, gastric disease, palpitations, rheumatic heart disease, limb pain, acute pericarditis, cerebral ischemia, rheumatic fever, and nausea and vomiting in pregnancy.

CLINICAL APPLICATIONS
Points 88.01, 88.02, and 88.03 are always combined as a Dao Ma for best results. These are some of the most frequently used points in the modern clinic due to the fact that most patients have some sort of heart Qi, or blood problem at the root of their disease. The number one killer in America is heart disease. There are many manifestations of heart disease, both in Western and Chinese medicine.

This three point unit is also exceptional to treat all types of spleen and stomach problems. Many patients have gastrointestinal issues exacerbating or causing their condition. Ailments such as stress, allergies, insomnia, and fatigue can all be caused by a poorly functioning digestive system.

These are some of the best points, if not the best points in the Tung system to treat any heart problem. They treat heart Qi deficiency, and heart Qi stagnation. I use them every day to treat circulation issues, edema in the legs, heart issues, tight chest sensation, and to tonify the blood.

Since this is the fire point and fire generates the earth, you can see why these points are so great for many digestion issues. They are also located in the thick muscles of the legs, which means they are related to the spleen, and digestion. In addition, they are on the ST channel, which goes through the digestive organs.

88.01, 88.02, and 88.03

These are the main points to treat edema caused by heart issues, and hypotension caused by heart conditions. These points are indicated for finger pain, but I do not use them much for that.

These are my favorite points to use on myself after a long week of working and standing on my feet all day. They treat chest palpitations from stress, disturbed sleep from too much work, fatigue, and edema in the lower legs from standing all day. These are the first points I do on myself when I feel this way.

There are many other listed indications that come from this root dysfunction. They are: heart diseases, pericardial pain, and pain on both sides of the heart, rheumatic heart disease, dizziness, vertigo, palpitations, gastric disease, limb pain, acute pericarditis, rheumatic fever, cerebral ischemia, four limb pain, gastritis, nausea and vomiting in pregnancy.

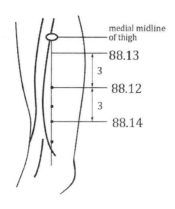

88.12
Ming Huang
Bright Yellow

88.13
Tian Huang
Heavenly Yellow

88.14
Qi Huang
Other Yellow

Three Upper Yellow
Dao Ma

TCM FUNCTIONS
Move, tonify, and sedate the liver organ, liver Qi, and liver blood. Stops wind, moves Qi and blood, and stops pain. Invigorates the KD, LV, and the HT.

REACTION AREA
Kidney (superficial depth). Liver (middle depth), Heart (deep level).

LOCATION AND NEEDLE TECHNIQUE
In the center of the medial aspect of the thigh. Perpendicular insertion, needle to the deep level to activate all 3 reaction areas.

88.12 is located on the midpoint of the inner thigh on the LV channel.
88.13 is located 3 cun proximal to 88.12 on the LV channel.
88.14 is located 3 cun distal to 88.12 on the LV channel

CLASSICAL INDICATIONS
Liver cirrhosis, hepatitis, body swelling, fatigue, back pain, chorea (e.g. Parkinsonism), leukemia, multiple sclerosis (especially with diplopia). Hepatocirrhosis, hepatitis, enlargement of bones, spinal periostitis, fatigue due to hypofunction of the Liver, soreness of the lower back, blurred vision, eye pain, hepatalgia, indigestion.

88.12, 88.13, and 88.14

CLINICAL APPLICATIONS
The main point is 88.12, and sometimes only this point is used. If 88.13 or 88.14 is used, always include 88.12, which is the most important point of the three. This is my favorite set of points. They are great for many things. The reason is that all our patients have liver issues, fatty, depressed, and stagnated livers. They have blood circulation problems, Qi and blood imbalances and stagnation. The heart and liver are the two most diseased organs in Western culture.

These points are clinically important for fatigue, eye issues, allergies, bone spurs, and liver pain. This is the most underused channel for the treatment of pain. It is also the most undertreated organ. It is the most undervalued pathology when it comes to patients with headaches, fertility, allergies, sleep problems, fatigue, pain, digestion, and "just not feeling right." These points should be used for more than just Western-defined cirrhosis of the liver, or the treatment of Hepatitis C.

These are some of the most important points I used on my wife to stop the early delivery of our son. They are amazing for miscarriage, which is also known as "slippery fetus."

I treated a patient with headaches that were not going away with "headache points," such as Da Bai (22.04) or 77.22 and 77.23. The reason the points were not working was that her headaches were caused by her menstrual cycle. The insertion of 88.12, 88.13, and 88.14 completely relieved her headache.

Another patient had fatigue. I tried many of the points indicated for fatigue in most Tung books. It did not work. The reason it did not work was that the fatigue was coming from too many Western medications, and too much alcohol consumption. Her liver was blocked, stagnated, and overworked. These points, 88.12, 88.13, and 88.14 relieved her headache immediately.

These points are like Ling Gu, an entire book could be written about them. They should be considered for any blood or Qi disease. They are also useful for any wind issue, shaking, tendon, or muscle disease. They are useful for odd diseases such as shaking diseases, like Parkinson's.

These are amazing points. They are clinically some of the most relevant and powerful points you can use in Western clinics. If I were to choose my top three points, this Dao Ma of 88.12, 88.13, and 88.14 would be included.

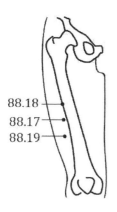

88.17
Si Ma Zhong
Rapid Horses Center

88.18
Si Ma Shang
Rapid Horses Upper

88.19
Si Ma Xia
Rapid Horses Lower

Three Upper Horses or
Si Ma Points Dao Ma

TCM FUNCTIONS
Tonifies lung Qi, dispels wind, damp, and phlegm, moves Qi and blood, and stops pain. Soothes and clears the liver.

LOCATION AND NEEDLE TECHNIQUE
Three cun anterior to the spot touched by the middle fingertip when one is standing with his hands at his sides. Perpendicular insertion between the ST and GB channels.

REACTION AREA
Liver, Lung

CLASSICAL INDICATIONS
Hypochondriac pain, back pain, sciatica and lower back pain due to hypofunction of the lungs, pneumonia, tuberculosis, chest and back pain due to injury, pleurisy, rhinitis, deafness, tinnitus, otitis, dermatitis, facial paralysis, congested eyes, asthma, breast pain (very effective), hemiplegia, psoriasis, dermatosis, and strain of the lower limbs. Pain on the lateral side of the ribs, sciatica, chest pain, pulmonary tuberculosis, conjunctivitis, breast pain, rhinitis, and dermatological disorders.

CLINICAL APPLICATION
Clinically, 88.17 is the main point in this Dao Ma, and it is always used. It is usually combined with 88.18 and 88.19.

This is a top point and top Dao Ma in the Tung system. This is the Five Zang line theory, which explains why it is so great for the lungs and skin, it is on the Five Zang line of the lung. This is more of an advanced concept of the Tung system, and one that will be more confusing than not for most, so I do not discuss it much.

88.17, 88.18 and 88.19

Master Tung said that unique to his system, all diseases were diseases of the five Zang organs, the heart, kidneys, lung, spleen, and liver. As long as we treated those five Zang, if they were diseased, disease would go away. In the Tung family system, they put lines down each limb, these lines on the body were given a "Zang," so each limb would have five lines. If there were points on these lines, such as 88.17, 88.18, or 88.19, they were on the lung line of the thigh, and thus would treat lung conditions.

Points 88.01, 88.02, and 88.03 are very effective for heart conditions. There are about 30 theories that explain why that is. One unique way that the Tung family would suggest is that those points, 88.01, 88.02, and 88.03, lie on the Zang line of the heart. That line, the heart Zang line, and any point on that line will treat the heart. In fact, all the points on that heart Zang line do treat the heart. This is very interesting, to say the least. Many theories can be attributed to a various people, but the Zang line, Zang disease and Zang pathology is unique to the Tung family.

These points are clinically relevant for sciatica, any type of chest pain, thoracic cavity pain, and any type of lung or skin issue. They treat any type of breathing, sinus, nose, diaphragm, and intercostal muscle issue. They should be your first choice to treat skin, nose, rib, and allergy issues.

These points are used a lot clinically to treat fibromyalgia, muscle weakness, general fatigue, numbness, and chronic overall pain.

They are the number one points for stuffy nose (the LU opens to the nose), the number one for allergies (the LU is the first affected organ), and they tonify Qi, because of the lung association. Since these points are located in a big muscle, they treat muscular problems.

I use these points a lot for sciatica. I treat the opposite side Ling Gu, Da Ba, San Cha San, with the same side 88.17, 88.18, and 88.19. This is a very effective point combination. It is also a great systemic treatment for fibromyalgia patients. This combination is used to treat hypothyroid and general fatigue. A wonderful combination is 88.12, 88.13, and 88.14 on one leg, with the other leg being 88.17, 88.18, and 88.19. This is a very powerful treatment.

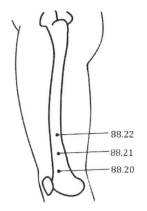

88.20
Xia Quan
Lower Spring

88.21
Zhong Quan
Center Spring

88.22
Shang Quan
Upper Spring

Three Springs Dao Ma

TCM FUNCTIONS
Expel and extinguish wind, open the channels and collaterals in the face. They are primarily indicated for diseases or issues on the GB and TW channels on the face.

REACTION AREA
Face, Lung

LOCATION AND NEEDLE TECHNIQUE
Perpendicular insertion, through the IT band. Touch the bone on insertion.

88.20 Two and a half cun superior to the knee joint, along the median line of the lateral thigh.
88.21 Two cun superior to 88.20.
88.22 Two cun superior to 88.21.

CLASSICAL INDICATIONS
Facial paralysis, facial tics, deviation of the eyes and mouth, tinnitus, poor hearing, and Bell's palsy.

CLINICAL APPLICATIONS
Points 88.20, 88.21, and 88.22 are always used together in a Dao Ma.

These points are not considered to be very popular, but in modern clinics they are extremely valuable points for most, if not all of your patients.

88.20, 88.21 and 88.22

The Ling Shu says that the GB is bone, so we need to needle down to the bone. The upper thigh images the face, both above and below the eyes. The GB is in charge of wind, shaking, tendons, and bone. Many patients have headaches on the frontal area, temples, and the side of the head, all of which are controlled by the GB. Frontal headaches are associated with Yang Ming, but there is a lot of GB involvement also.

This Dao Ma group is remarkable for any issue in the upper face, in particular when that issue is on the GB, or TW channels on the face, or for wind. They are remarkable for GB or TW headaches, TMJ pain, eye tics, Bell's palsy, and trigeminal neuralgia. They are not effective for tinnitus, but they treat any other ear problem, and temporal side head problem. I use them a lot for ear pain, ear stuffiness, ear blockages, ear swelling, but not tinnitus.

I have used these points to treat idiopathic large arteritis in one patient. I have also used them to treat hydrocephalus and many head traumas.

As long as my patient has time and is welling to allow me to needle their thighs, these points are my preferred choice to treat head problems.

As a general rule, for chronic conditions I prefer to treat the legs. Master Tung used the legs in general for chronic issues and clinically I agree. All the points are fantastic but the points on the legs (feet, lower legs, upper legs) are all so powerful. They are, to me, the best of the best.

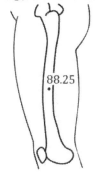
Zhong Jiu Li - Center Nine Miles

88.25

88.25
Zhong Jiu Li
Center Nine Miles

TCM FUNCTIONS
Courses the wind, clears heat, clears the head and opens the portals, sharpens hearing, frees the channels and quickens the connecting vessels. Moves LV Qi, breaks stagnation, clears blockages, and treats bones and sinews. Invigorates Kidney Qi, courses the liver, soothes the heart, and quiets the Shen.

REACTION AREA
All four limbs, Lung

LOCATION AND NEEDLE TECHNIQUE
This point is located in the same location as the TCM point GB 31. It can be located by finding the middle of the femur on the GB channel, or where the patient's finger tips touch the IT band on the GB Channel. Clinically I prefer to find it by finding the midway point on the femur on the GB channel. Perpendicular insertion, through the IT band to the lateral side of the femur. You must insert the needle through to touch the bone.

CLASSICAL INDICATIONS
There are many other indications for this point. They depend on the root cause and include the following indications: Back pain, lower back pain, lumbar vertebral pain, hemiplegia, facial paralysis, neck pain, and dizziness, distending feeling in the eyes, numbness of the hand and arm and leg. Pain in the lateral side of the thigh, migraine headaches, cervical spondylosis, facial pain, tinnitus, leg or knee pain, bone spurs, and lack of strength in the nerves.

88.25
Zhong Jiu Li
Center Nine Miles

CLINICAL APPLICATIONS

Since this point is located on the upper thigh and Western patients often do not disrobe, this point is not used as often as it could be. It is amazing. I know that it might seem difficult to some acupuncturists to treat the upper thighs or the upper arms. However, the upper legs and upper arms are quite clinically valuable.

Most, if not all, of our patients have stress, pain, and sleep issues, due to many factors. Point 88.25 is the best point to treat all of these issues. This point should be needled on the lateral side of the femur, it is very important that you touch the femur. This point is like 77.01, 77.02, and 77.03. If you do not tap the bone, it is only 50% effective.

This point is one of my top points to treat all sorts of head issues, the face, eyes, ears, TMJ, headaches, teeth, or jaw pain. If the problem is located on the head, this is the first point I consider.

It is also the first point to consider to treat any pathology related to wind. If there is any tendon, shaking, bone spur, pain, or trauma, this point should be used. The GB treats the LV and tendons, which treats wind and shaking. It also treats the bones and pain.

It is the premiere point to treat when it comes to weird diseases. According to the Classics, "wind is the source of 10,000 diseases." This point is the most frequently used point in my clinic. It rarely lets me down, it rarely fails to work as expected.

In just one day in clinic, I used this point to treat:

- Stress, hypertension, and Liver Qi stagnation
- Overall wellness and anti-aging – 2 patients
- ALS, back pain, and peripheral neuropathy
- Elbow pain and arm pain
- Lower back pain at the PSIS, from long term degeneration and spurs
- Jaw pain and temporal headaches
- Stress and insomnia, Liver Qi stagnation, Heart Qi deficiency, Spleen damp
- Systemic pain in an Afghanistan war veteran with PTSD
- Neck pain from degeneration after a car accident, adhesions, and scar tissue
- Lower back pain from unknown causes in three different patients.
- General arthritis

88.25
Zhong Jiu Li
Center Nine Miles

- Sleep problems and neck pain
- Fatigue and general aches and pains, and fibromyalgia that "just flared up"
- General autoimmune diseases, digestion issues, and histamine release problems associated with the intestines.
- Stress in four different patients, and SAD (seasonal affective disorder)
- Allergies
- Headache on the entire head
- Jaw pain and TMJ
- All legs and arms hurt after falling down while hunting

In one day, with 30 patients, this point was used on 27 patients for a multitude of reasons. You can see the depth and richness of this point, and the theories that support it clinically. With so many indication, it helps to think of 88.25 for:

- It is a top point in the Tung system. It is in the top 2-3 most used points.
- It is amazing for: Pain, insomnia, stress (GB/HT for sleep, GB/LV for stress.)
- I often bleed the ear apex and needle 88.25 for sleep or stress, with any underlying pathology.
- Top point for bone spurs, TMJ, facial issues, eye, ear, mouth, problems, because the GB controls the bone per the Ling Shu.
- It is the top point for systemic pain, due to the reaction area of the four limbs. I will often combine it with Ling Gu, and sit back and see what heals or what does not improve.
- It is the top point for any Wind condition, it is called the "wind market."
- Top point for trigeminal neuralgia, Bell's palsy, and any head problem. It is even better if it is a temporal head problem.
- If in doubt, use 88.25, it is that amazing.
- It is wonderful for peripheral neuropathy issues.
- It was even said that to learn Tung acupuncture "fast and easy" you should just use two points for pain. The first point was on the opposite side of the pain, in the exact spot of the pain. Add 88.25 on the same side. This was said to be the fastest way to learn Tung style pain treatment method, and it is effective the majority of the time.

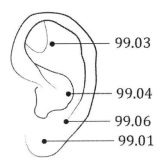

99.01
Er Huan
Ear Ring
Intoxication from alcohol and vomiting.
In the center of the ear lobe.

99.03
Hou Er
Fire Ear
Heart failure, knee, and limb pain.
In the middle of the outer border of the antihelix.

99.04
Tu Er
Earth Ear
Neurasthenia, polycythemia, high fever, and diabetes.
In the center of the cavity of the concha.

99.06
Shui Er
Water Ear
Kidney deficiency, pain on both sides of the lower back, and abdominal distension.
At the lower end of the outer border of antihelix.

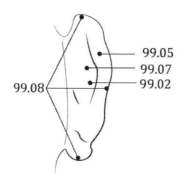

99.02
Mu Er
Wood Ear

Liver pain, hepatomegaly, hepatocirrhosis, and fatigue due to deficiency in the Liver, and chronic strangury.

Longitudinally, 0.3 cun below the middle transverse branch of the dorsal auricular artery of the posterior side of the ear.

99.05
Jin Er
Wood Ear

Sciatica due to hypofunction of the Lung, lumbar vertebra bending and allergic common cold.

One third of a cun superior to Shui Er (99.06).

99.07
Er Bei
Back of Ear

Pharyngitis and tonsillitis.

About 0.33 cun above Mu Er (99.03).

Bleed the point with a three-edged needle.

99.08
Er San
Ear Three

Cholera, migraine, common cold, and tonsillitis.

On the outer border of the helix of the ear.

Bleed the points with a three-edged needle.

99.00 Ear Points

From a Tung perspective, one of the top 10 Tung treatments is to bleed the ear apex. I do this quite often to treat allergies, systemic pain, shingles, stye in the eye, hypertension, stress, insomnia, a hangover, motion sickness, night sweats, lower back pain, common cold, and migraine headaches. It is a remarkable treatment to bleed, and or needle the ear apex.

Why does this work? Bloodletting is an art in itself. One third of all Master Tung patients were bled. I have bled thousands of patients. In India, we noticed that acupuncture alone was not enough to treat chronic pain patients. After one month of treatment, things started to turn around with them. We would not do acupuncture until after we bled them first. If a patient had a chronic disease, they were always bled first. This dramatically increased our results. I would bleed over fifty patients a day in India. This does not mean that we took a lot of blood from them. Just a few drops, or perhaps a tablespoon of blood was enough.

The other part of the ear that I bled a lot is the back of the ear. It is important to bleed all the visible veins on the back of the ear. The ear relates to the Kidney, all the yang channels run through the ear. The heart opens to the ear, via the Su Wen. The heart and kidney communicate. The GB, Shao Yang channels, all around the ear, the BL or Tai Yang channels go to the ear.

The heart opens the orifices, controls sweat, and controls fluids. Liver Yang and Liver fire rise up to the ears. The heart and kidney meet at the ear and are the "fire and water." There are so many things, channels, ideas, theories, and relationships that happen around the ear. It is a very powerful thing to treat.

Point 99.07 is a special point, because you can needle or bleed all the veins on the back of the ear for dermatology, migraine headaches, TMJ, dizziness, nausea, shock, seasickness, and any head problem.

Clinically, I will needle the ear apex and or needle the back of the ear, assuming there are visible veins. I do this every day in my clinic to treat stress, sleep, systemic pain, systemic stagnation, headaches, jaw problems, and dizziness. This is also good for patients who say they feel out of sorts, under the weather, feel down or tired, or just not right.

117

99.00 Ear Points

I use the ear every day for patients with a common cold, the sniffles, and any type of excess yang, fire, heat, or inflammatory condition. They are points not to be dismissed.

Don't forget that the ear apex is a top 10 point in the Tung system. You can needle it, but I suggest you bleed it. It is a shame that bloodletting is not a more common practice. I think most people would be amazed beyond what they think is possible, with the instant and miraculous healing.

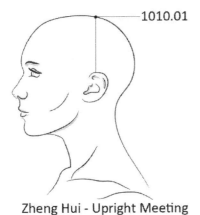
Zheng Hui - Upright Meeting

1010.01
Zheng Hui
Upright Meeting

TCM FUNCTIONS
Expels wind, treats liver wind, suppresses liver yang, clears the spirit, discharges blazing heat from the Yang channels, and lifts fallen Yang and Qi.

REACTION AREA
Brain, Cerebral nerve

LOCATION AND NEEDLE TECHNIQUE
Located at Du 20. Perpendicular insertion. If this point hurts on insertion, withdraw the needle and re-insert. The pain is due to the needle tip hitting a hair follicle. Re-insertion will fix this. Insert .1 to .3 cun deep.

CLASSICAL INDICATIONS
Hemiplegia, fatigue, tremors, infantile convulsions, eye and mouth deviation (from stroke), aphasia due to stroke, dysfunction of nervous system, stroke sequellae, cerebral palsy.

CLINICAL APPLICATIONS
This point is located at Du 20. This point is used clinically for pain under the chin, Ren 1 or Du 1 pain, and heel pain. It is also often used in conjunction with Si Shen Cong. From a Master Tung perspective, this is often combined with 1010.05 and 1010.06 to treat stress.

There are not a lot of points in the Tung system that treat stress, so this point is used a lot for that. I will typically combine 1010.01, 1010.05, and 1010.06 with 1010.08 as the top four points from Master Tung for stress.

1010.01
Zheng Hui
Upright Meeting

In my opinion, the weakness of the Tung system is in treating emotional indications. Master Tung did not see a lot of stress, anxiety, or depression the way it manifests in our clinics today. Hence he does not have a lot of points with the indication of stress. I have treated tens of thousands of patients overseas who live in rural areas. The term stress does not really exist in these communities. In India, for example, out of 8,000 cases I treated stress twice. Master Tung has more points to treat polio and tuberculosis, which were the most common diseases of his time.

The other big clinical indication is for yang rising and liver wind. These points are used a lot for non-essential tremors, shaking, and they balance any type of brain disorder, because of the reaction area of the brain. This point treats any condition arising from liver yang, or liver wind, such as stroke sequellae which could be aphasia, or hemiplegia. Other indications are fatigue, deviation of the eye and mouth, infantile convulsions, Parkinson's, cerebral palsy, tics, tremor of the limbs, and dysfunction of the nervous system.

I find this point to be extremely effective to treat hemiplegia, as long as you can treat it within 30 days of the event, preferably the next day. When I treat patients overseas, patients are often brought to me the day after their stroke. In cases like this, the results are fast and amazing. The more time that has elapsed since the event, the harder it is to treat it.

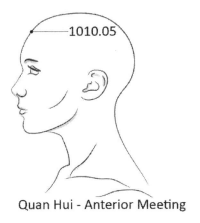
Quan Hui - Anterior Meeting

1010.05
Qian Hui
Anterior Meeting

TCM FUNCTIONS
Expels wind heat, liver wind, sedates liver yang, clears the spirit, discharges blazing heat from the Yang channels, and raises sunken Yang and Qi.

REACTION AREA
Brain

LOCATION AND NEEDLE TECHNIQUE
One and a half cun anterior to Zheng Hui (1010.01). Perpendicular insertion. If insertion is painful, withdraw the needle and re-insert. Sometimes the needle hits a hair follicle, re-inserting the needle will fix it. Insert the needle 0.1-0.3 cun deep.

CLASSICAL INDICATIONS
Dizziness, blurred vision, distending feeling of the head, and neurasthenia.

CLINICAL APPLICATIONS
This is point is always used with 1010.01 and 1010.06 for stress and brain disorders please see 1010.01 for further details.

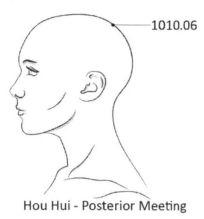

Hou Hui - Posterior Meeting

**1010.06
Hou Hui
Posterior Meeting**

TCM FUNCTIONS
Expels wind, liver wind, lowers liver yang, clears the spirit, discharges blazing heat from the yang channels, and lifts fallen yang and Qi.

REACTION AREA
Brain, Spine

LOCATION AND NEEDLE TECHNIQUE
Located 1.6 cun posterior to Zheng Hui (1010.01). Perpendicular insertion. If insertion is painful, withdraw the needle and re-insert. Sometimes the needle hits a hair follicle, re-inserting the needle will fix it. Insert the needle 0.1-0.3 cun deep.

CLASSICAL INDICATIONS
Bone tuberculosis, dizziness, headaches, spinal pain, and stroke.

CLINICAL APPLICATIONS
This point can be used clinically for general bone pain. It is also effective for random headaches, if they are caused by liver wind, liver yang rising, wind heat or cold, or liver Qi stagnation. It also treats the manifestations of wind stroke, including aphasia.

I always use 1010.01, 1010.05, and 1010.06 together as a Dao Ma for stress, insomnia, and to treat cranial nerve dysfunctions such as shaking or essential tremors. An essential tremor is also called a benign essential tremor. It is a brain disorder that causes a part of your body to shake uncontrollably. The shaking is called tremors.

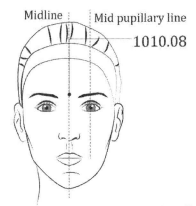

Midline | Mid pupillary line

1010.08

Zhen Jing - Tranquil and Still

1010.08
Zhen Jing
Tranquil and Still

TCM FUNCTIONS
Calms the Shen, sedates the spirit, and quiets the heart. It is very effective for any weakness, sleep issue, or shaking of the limbs due to stress. It clears the Shen and brain, and is helpful for nightmares or disturbed sleep.

REACTION AREA
Brain

LOCATION AND NEEDLE TECHNIQUE
One third of a cun above the midpoint between the eyebrows. Insert the needle subcutaneously towards the nose with a depth of 0.1-0.2 cun. Pinch the skin a little and raise the skin from the forehead, insert the needle gently. This is important, because if inserted this way, you will not bruise your patient.

CLASSICAL INDICATIONS
Mental and stress disorders, tremor of limbs, weakness of legs, insomnia, nightmares, restless legs, and limb paralysis.

CLINICAL APPLICATIONS
This point is similar to Yin Tang. It is very effective and is often combined in clinic with 1010.01, 1010.05, and 1010.06 to treat stress, insomnia, depression, anxiety, Liver Qi stagnation, and Liver Yang rising. I usually combine 1010.01, 1010.05, 1010.06, and 1010.08 as a four point Dao Ma for depression. I rarely use 1010.08 alone.

A nice way to increase the effectiveness of this point is to add TCM point An Mian, and TCM ear point Ear Shen Men. I use this as one my main points for stress reduction in the clinic. This is also one my favorite points for treating the brain (because of the reaction area). I use it for such conditions as brain trauma, swelling, irritation, and inflammation etc.

Ma Jin Shui - Horse Metal Water

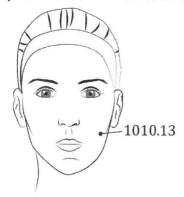

1010.13

1010.13
Ma Jin Shui
Horse Metal Water

TCM FUNCTIONS
The Chinese name for 1010.13 means to "free up, free going," and it means "water kidney." The point name tells you what it does. The full combined name means "moving Qi and rooting the kidney."

It tonifies the Kidneys, regulates Qi, tonifies Kidney Qi, disinhibits urination, dispels damp, frees blockages, and clears heat.

REACTION AREA
Kidney, Lung

LOCATION AND NEEDLE TECHNIQUE
Located in the depression beneath the lower border of the zygomatic bone, directly below the outer canthus. Insert the needle 0.1-0.3 cun deep. Perpendicular insertion. Since you are treating the KD, which is bone, it is better if you tap the bone. Tapping the bone increases the effectiveness of this point.

CLASSICAL INDICATIONS
Nephritis, kidney stones, lower back pain, sciatica, chest pain, regulating free flow of Qi and water metabolism. Promoting the kidney and moving Qi. Regulating the kidney and prostate.

CLINICAL APPLICATIONS
This point is usually combined with 1010.14 to form a Dao Ma. Point 1010.13 treats the kidneys, and 1010.14 treats the bladder. However, since the functions are so similar, it is helpful to use them together. They are quite effective to treat lower back pain from kidney issues, including kidney stones. They also treat bladder issues, including bladder stones.

These points are used to treat kidney stones, nephritis, lower back pain, sciatica, chest pain affected upon breathing, prostate issues, male sexual issues, edema, and urinary tract infections.

1010.13
Ma Jin Shui
Horse Metal Water

This point is located at SI 18, and although Master Tung does not use the same indications as this point, they do have one common link. This point is on the SI channel, and the SI clears turbid damp, this is the common thread. Many of the Master Tung indications are for "stuck turbid damp fluid," which these points treat.

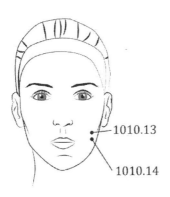

Ma Kuai Shui - Horse Fast Water

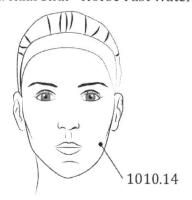

1010.14

1010.14
Ma Kuai Shui
Horse Fast Water

TCM FUNCTIONS

The Chinese name of this point means to "speed up, speed up water." It is important for the bladder. It speeds up water, when the bladder is full of urine. It is always combined with 1010.13.

Tonifies the Kidneys, regulates Qi, tonifies Kidney Qi, disinhibits urination, dispels damp, frees blockages, and clears heat. Point 1010.14 is more focused on treating the bladder, and 1010.13 is focused on the kidneys.

REACTION AREA

Kidney, Bladder

LOCATION AND NEEDLE TECHNIQUE

Located .4 cun below Ma Jin Shui, 1010.13. Insert perpendicular to the face, the needle is inserted straight into the point.

CLASSICAL INDICATIONS

Bladder stones, cystitis, frequent urination, lumbar pain, and rhinitis.

CLINICAL APPLICATIONS

This point is almost always used in combination with 1010.14. These points are very effective for kidney and bladder problems. They also treat back pain that is located near the kidneys or originating in the kidneys. They can also be used for urinary tract infections, although Chinese herbs are the preferred treatment.

When patients have kidney or bladder pain that refers to the back, or they have kidney stones or bladder stones that cause back pain, these points are used.

These points can be used to treat any indication that can be treated by moving Qi, promoting Kidney function, and improving water metabolism. I use these points in my clinic frequently for prostate issues and they are very effective.

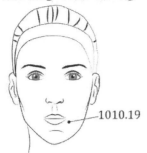

Shui Tong - Water Through

1010.19

1010.19
Shui Tong
Water Through

TCM FUNCTIONS
KIDNEY INDICATIONS
Kidney yin and yang deficiency, kidney weakness, adrenal fatigue (kidney yang deficiency). This point supplements the kidneys, secures essence, courses the channels and regulates Qi. It regulates qi and blood circulation.

LUNG INDICATIONS
Dispels wind, transforms phlegm, rectifies the lung, and suppresses coughing. Clears the upper burner from wind, damp and phlegm, tonifies lung Qi.

REACTION AREA
Kidney

LOCATION AND NEEDLE TECHNIQUE
Half cun below the corner of the mouth. See 1010.20 for needling technique, I almost always needle these two points together with one needle.

CLASSICAL INDICATIONS
Lower back pain, acute lumbar sprain, vertigo, dizziness, fatigue, difficulty breathing, and asthma.

CLINICAL APPLICATIONS
This point is combined with 1010.20. Please refer to 1010.20 for clinical applications. There are many symptoms that can arise from a poorly functioning adrenal, kidney and lung system. I use these points frequently in clinic because they treat the root and the branch.

Some common manifestations for this point are: Lower back pain, acute lumbar sprain, vertigo, dizziness, fatigue, coughing, dyspnea, asthma, chest pain, constriction, or tightness. It tonifies the kidneys, treats fibromyalgia, adrenal fatigue, low hormones, and weak breathing due to a lung Qi deficiency.

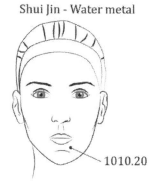

Shui Jin - Water metal

1010.20

1010.20
Shui Jin
Water Metal

TCM FUNCTIONS
KIDNEY INDICATIONS
Kidney yin and yang deficiency, kidney weakness, adrenal fatigue (kidney yang deficiency). Supplements the kidneys, secures the essence, courses the channels and regulates Qi. Regulates Qi and blood circulation. Secures the Qi, and the breath.

LUNG INDICATIONS
Dispels wind, transforms phlegm, rectifies the lung, and suppresses coughing. Clears the upper burner and Lung Qi.

REACTION AREA
Kidney

LOCATION AND NEEDLE TECHNIQUE
Located a half cun medial and a 45 degree angle to Shui Tong (1010.19). Note: Always thread one needle from 1010.19 to 1010.20.

See 1010.20 for technique. If you prefer, you can use two needles. Insert one needle perpendicularly into 1010.19, and one needle into 1010.20. The easier and faster way is to use one needle threaded from 1010.20 to 1010.19.

Start at 1010.20 and pinch the skin a bit, you do not want to drive the needle through the lip and into the mouth. By pinching the skin, it gives you a little skin that is superficial, that makes it easier to insert. Gently slide the needle at a 45 degree angle up towards 1010.19. The needles should look like they are at a 45 degree angle to the mouth when you are done.

CLASSICAL INDICATIONS
Lower back pain, acute lumbar sprain, vertigo, dizziness, fatigue, difficulty breathing, and asthma.

1010.20
Shui Jin
Water Metal

CLINICAL APPLICATIONS

Points 1010.19 and 1010.20 are some of the more well-known Tung points. They are used for lower back pain, but it is important to distinguish what type of back pain. It is back pain that involves the kidney organ, which is located in the area of T10-T12. This point is very effective for lower back pain in the *muscles* of the lower back. It can be described as a "band" around the lower back. When patients say they have sore and achy back muscles, these are the points to use to treat them.

Other clinically useful indications are any lung or breathing problem, any lung or kidney issue, cough, or asthma issue. They are extremely effective for these issues. They are the best choice to treat asthma and allergies.

This point is combined with 1010.19. There are so many manifestations that can originate from poorly functioning adrenals, kidneys and the lung system. I use these points often in the clinic, because patients often have this root and branch issue. I commonly use these points for any breathing issue, lung related asthma, or cough.

Some commonly seen manifestations are: lower back pain, acute lumbar sprain, vertigo, dizziness, fatigue, coughing, dyspnea, and asthma. Chest pain, constriction, and tightness. Kidney weakness, fibromyalgia, adrenal fatigue, low hormone levels, and weak breathing due to weak lungs.

The indications for this point are due to the effect it has on the lungs or kidneys, and the adrenal system.

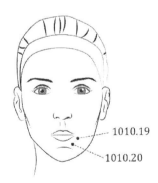

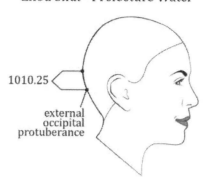

Zhou Shui - Prefecture Water

1010.25

external
occipital
protuberance

1010.25
Zhou Shui
Prefecture Water

TCM FUNCTIONS
Treats the bones and sinews on the lower Du channel, from L4 to S4. They move qi and blood in the Du channel in the L4-S4 area. They stop pain, numbness, and weakness in the lower back, and also treat issues originating in this area.

REACTION AREA
Kidney

LOCATION AND NEEDLE TECHNIQUE
Use one needle threaded down from the second point to the first point of this two point unit. The first point is just superior to the EOP (external occipital protuberance). The second point is .8 cun superior to the first point. Insert the needle .8 cun. There are 10 fen in 1 cun. I think the easiest way to think of needling is to start your needle at Du 18 and needle down to Du 17.

CLASSICAL INDICATIONS
Pain on the spine, paralysis of the legs.

CLINICAL APPLICATIONS

These points treat sciatica, spinal stenosis, compression, bone spurs, foramen narrowing, disc degeneration, disc compression, radiculopathy, piriformis syndrome, ischial tuberosity pain, sacral pain, and PSIS pain.

About 100 different back problems originate in the area of L4 and S4. To acupuncturists, it is all the same, we treat the root, and the root is the spine and the joints of the spine. We need to treat the Du channel, which is the root. The disease manifestation is for Western medicine to define and placate, but never heal.

1010.25
Zhou Shui
Prefecture Water

This is one of the most commonly used Tung points to treat back pain. It is extremely effective to treat lower back pain on the sacrum. The external occipital protuberance images the sacrum. This point treats the area from L5 to S4. It is most effective to treat pain on the Du channel.

Insert the needle .8 cun to 1 cun superior to the EOP and thread the needle down over the EOP. This will treat L4-5 and S1-4. I have seen patients with pain on a scale of 7/10, with spinal pain from epidurals or surgeries get up and be instantly pain free with one treatment. This was my first one needle treatment in India. A patient had an epidural for childbirth seven years prior to her treatment. She had pain every day since that time. Her pain vanished after one needle was threaded down the EOP. The pain never returned.

The trick to inserting this point painlessly is to use your left hand, or whatever hand is your non-needle hand. Once you insert the needle, the needle will want to bury itself and go toward the skull. Use your non needle hand and press your finger just at the base of the needle tip just after inserting it in the scalp. As you press just proximal to the tip of the needle, it will make the tip of the needle bend just a bit. This little bit of bend will make sure the needle is angled away from the skull, and it will bury itself in the scalp.

As you insert the needle downward, toward the EOP, just continue to press the needle proximal to the tip of the needle, this will allow the needle to remain more superficial on insertion.

You know that you have inserted your needle correctly if it just slides easily down the skull. If you are pushing too hard, have to force the needle, and it is getting stuck, the needle is too deep. Insert the needle more superficially so it glides between the skull and the scalp, down to the point. Just like butter. It is a very smooth insertion.

This is one of the few points that will alleviate pain in patients with foramen narrowing. This is a very difficult condition to treat with acupuncture or herbs. This condition typically requires surgery, but this point is amazing to treat it. It is typically used to treat the narrowing of the foramen in the lower back.

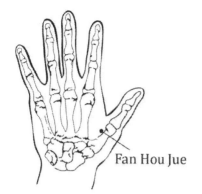

Fan Hou Jue

Cutting Opposite and Behind

TCM FUNCTIONS
Moves Qi and blood, stops pain in the upper back at TW 15, GB 21, SI 14, SI 15, and BL 21 area. Move Qi and blood to relieve pain in the shoulder area. Tonifies the Lungs.

REACTION AREA
Lung

LOCATION AND NEEDLING TECHNIQUE
This point is located one cun distal to Ling Gu. The needle is inserted next to the thumb bone. This point is on the dorsal side of the hand. Point 22.01 is located on the palmar side of this point.

CLASSICAL INDICATIONS
This point is great for stiff upper back and shoulders, and for shoulder pain. It is most famous for shoulder pain, and it treats any type. The etiology of the shoulder pain is irrelevant. This is the first choice to treat shoulder pain. This point usually clears all channels and relieves the pain. If necessary, additional points can be added if this does not resolve all the pain.

It also treats the upper back due to the fact that it is on the LI and LU channels. The LU treats the BL, which covers a large area of the upper back. It treats the LI channel via the Jing Jin theory, which treats the trapezius muscles and subscapularis. These two channels treat many channels in the back. The thumb joint images the upper back and shoulder area.

The Tung system does not have many points for the upper back and GB 21 area. Although 22.01 and 22.02 are very popular for upper back pain in the area of GB 21, I find that Fan Hou Jue is much better at treating pain in the area of GB 21, TW 15, BL 21, BL 22, BL 23, SI 14, and SI 15.

Fan Hou Jue

I usually combine Fan Hou Jue with Ling Gu. Most Tung teachers would say that you always combine Ling Gu with Da Bai. In my experience, I prefer to combine Fan Hou Jue with Ling Gu, rather than combining Ling Gu with Da Bai. I have come to this conclusion after using these points combined in this way for 10,000 treatments. I believe that the famous Ling Gu and Da Bai combination should be changed to the "new idea for modern clinics of combining Ling Gu and Fan Hou Jue."

A common point combination is to make a "Ling Gu Triangle." This is Ling Gu, Da Bai, and Fan Hou Jue. These three points treat a host of problems and complaints. I use it 20 times a day, it is that effective.

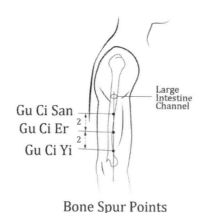

Bone Spur Points

Gu Ci Yi Er San

Bone Spur Points

Gu Ci Er
Gu Ci Yi
Gu Ci San

– Bone Spur One, Two, and Three

TCM FUNCTIONS
These points move Qi and blood and stop pain on the entire Du channel, in particular mid thoracic and lower back from T12 to S4. They strengthen Kidney Qi. They free the channels, the Du and KD, and regulate stagnation.

Moves Qi and blood and stop pain on the entire Du channel, in particular the mid thoracic and lower back (T12-S4). Treats Kidney deficiency. Frees the channels (the Du and KD) and harmonizes constriction. The Kidneys govern the bones, and they treat bone Bi syndrome.

REACTION AREA
Liver, Kidney. (Gu Ci San is listed as Liver only)

LOCATION AND NEEDLE TECHNIQUE
These points are a little unusual to insert.
Hold the arm with your fingers, you will feel the humerus bone. The humerus does not go straight up, it is angled slightly as you move upward. Not realizing that the humerus is not straight can make you miss the points. The needles *must* tap the humerus on the LI channel. If you do not tap the bone, your points will only be 50 percent effective.

LI 12 is the first point, Gu Ci Yi
Gu Ci Er is 2 cun proximal from Gu Ci YI
Gu Ci San is 2 cun proximal from Gu Ci Er
All three points are on the LI channel

Gu Ci Yi Er San
Bone Spur Points

CLASSICAL INDICATIONS
Bone spurs, sour pain of the vertebrae, traumatic injury of the vertebrae.

CLINICAL APPLICATIONS
These points are more effective than Ling Gu to treat lower back pain. They are extremely effective, and they are less painful for patients. These three points treat the upper, middle, and lower part of the spine. Whereas Ling Gu is just one point and it treats lower back pain. The Bone Spur points are used 70% of the time, and Ling Gu is used 30% of the time. They are extremely effective points.

These points are effective due to the LI treating the KD relationship of the back. Back pain usually manifests as muscular pain. The root originates at the spine, due to a compression or degeneration. If you can treat the spine, you can resolve back pain. These points treat the spine and they cover a larger area than Ling Gu. Ling Gu can be painful for patients and covers a more focused area. There is no equal to the Bone Spur Points. The Kidneys govern the bones, and they treat bone Bi syndrome.

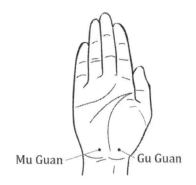

Gu Guan
Bone Gate

Mu Guan
Wood Gate

TCM FUNCTIONS
These points are used to treat Bi pain syndrome, in particular Damp Bi pain. They clear obstruction in the channels and collaterals.

REACTION AREA
Both points are Kidney and Lung

LOCATION AND NEEDLE TECHNIQUE
Mu Guan is located at the base of the palm, .5 cun distal to the pisiform bone. Gu Guan is located at the base of the palm, in the depression .5 cun distal to the scaphoid bone. Perpendicular insertion, make sure you touch the bone on insertion. We are treating bone pain, so we must touch or tap the bone with the needle.

CLASSICAL INDICATIONS
Swelling of the joints, rheumatoid arthritis, bone swelling, and heel pain.

CLINICAL APPLICATIONS
Mu Guan and Gu Guan are great points that are taught by Dr. Tan and included in his Twelve and Twelve book. They are also included in Master Tung's books. Dr. Tan even teaches a point called Zhong Guan, which means that it is located between Mu Guan and Gu Guan. This is a three point unit to treat bone swelling. I usually just use two points, but sometimes three points are indicated.

These points are clinically effective for systemic bone swelling, systemic arthritis, and damp Bi pain. They are also extremely effective to treat heel pain, instep pain, and plantar fasciitis, due to the image of the hand for the foot. I frequently use these points in conjunction with other points for rheumatoid arthritis pain, or osteoarthritis pain. These points clear pain all over the body.

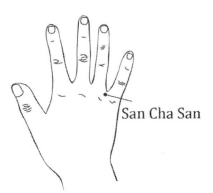

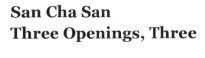
San Cha San
Three Openings, Three

San Cha San

TCM FUNCTIONS
Tonifies the spleen and kidney. Releases the exterior and expels wind. Moves Qi and blood, and stops pain. Opens the channels and collaterals.

REACTION AREA
Spleen, Kidney

LOCATION AND NEEDLE TECHNIQUE
With your free hand, pull the skin a bit to make the skin tight, not too tight though, just a little. This will remove the slack in the skin, and when you insert the needle, it will be easy to insert. Stop. Wait a few seconds, then continue with your insertion. If you slow down on the insertion, the needle will easily glide back into the joint space. I needle this on five year olds, and 100 year olds, 20 times a day. Out of all these treatments, only once a week does someone complain that it hurts. It is not painful to the patient, this point is easy to insert, just slow down and do not fear inserting the needle. Insert 1 to 1.5 cun deep.

CLASSICAL INDICATIONS
Knee joint pain, acute lumbar sprain, and diseases of the five sense organs. It also strengthens the heart. Common cold, headaches, shoulder pain, tinnitus, palpitations, hives, leg pain, fatigue, spleen Qi issues. It opens the five orifices of the face, treats heavy eyes, sweating, weak muscles, and thigh pain.

San Cha San

CLINICAL APPLICATIONS

This is one of the top 10 points in the Tung system. All the indications are extremely clinically effective, and appropriate.

I use this point every day, on most of my patients to treat neck pain, back pain, fatigue, opening the orifices of the face, common cold, itching conditions, weak and heavy eyes, shoulder pain, headaches, ear problems (although it is not great for tinnitus), heart conditions, and palpitations. It is an amazing point that I recommend everyone learn how to use.

I use San Cha San for back pain caused by kidney issues, because the TW treats the KD. Pain caused by dampness (spleen is the fourth finger in Tung palmar diagnosis). San Cha San is said to be TW 2, TW 3, TW 4, 22.06, 22.07, SI 3, SI 4, 22.08, and 22.09 all rolled into one. That is why there are so many indications for this one point. I will typically defer to San Cha San over using 22.06 and 22.07. They both cover the same points, but San Cha San covers more area, and thus has more, and more clinically useful indications.

The most famous point combination in the Tung system is Ling Gu, Da Bai, Zhong Bai, and 22.06. I would suggest a better combination for back pain is simply Ling Gu and San Cha San. This is much more powerful, and one fewer point to treat. In my opinion, San Cha San should be included with Ling Gu (22.05), 88.25, 77.18, and 77.08 as the most commonly used points in the Tung system.

San Cha San is extremely effective to treat any head issue, including red eyes, stuffy nose, congested sinuses, blocked ears, Qi stagnation in the face, wind attacking the face, and Bell's palsy. I often default to San Cha San for any issue of the upper neck, head, and face. It is one of the most important points for fatigue. I prefer it over other popular Tung points for fatigue. It has special indications for the heart, chest, fibromyalgia, chronic pain, and allergies. These all seem to be unrelated, but as you delve into the theory and application of these points, you will find they are all related.

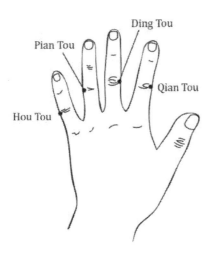

Tou Points

Hou Tou
Pian Tou
Ding Tou
Qian Tou

TCM FUNCTIONS
Move Qi and blood in the head. They resolve the exterior on the head, course wind, and clear the head.

LOCATION AND NEEDLE TECHNIQUE
Qian Tou and Ding Tou are needled in the direction of the little finger.
Pian Tou and Hou Tou are needled in the direction of the thumb.

All needles are perpendicular and the points are located where the pink and white skin meet. The needle is inserted to the bone. We are treating the skull, brain and head, so our needle must touch the bone to be effective.

CLINICAL APPLICATIONS
These points are remarkable for headaches. Each point treats a specific part of the head, but I have found it is better to just treat all four points to make sure the headache is relieved completely. If you just use one point, you might not address all aspects of the pain.

These four points are in the top three to four point combinations to treat headaches. They are very effective to treat headaches from Qi and blood disturbances in the head. They are not the best points if the headache is caused by something else, such as a hormonal imbalance, high blood pressure, or if a patient is going through detox. They will help, but the true strength of these points is when someone has a headache that originates on the head.

Tou Points

If you want to use one Tou point at a time, these are the locations they treat:

Qian Tou – Frontal headaches
Ding Tou – Vertex headaches
Pian Tou – Parietal headaches
Hou Tou – Occipital headaches

Headaches are commonly misdiagnosed. If the pain does not originate on the head or brain area, we need to consider where it does originate. Some common causes of headaches are hormonal imbalances, allergies, intestinal fungus, toxicity, stress, kidneys, heart, spleen dampness, gallbladder dysfunction, acid reflux, thyroid malfunction, constipation, or any other idiopathic cause. I love these points to treat headaches, but please remember to consider the root cause in your treatment.

Xiao Jie

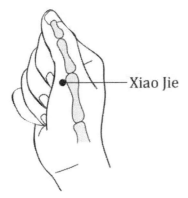

Xiao Jie

TCM FUNCTIONS
This point treats the ankle, foot, shoulder, and back. It moves Qi and blood to stop pain, and courses and clears the channels.

MIDDLE JIAO
Harmonizes the stomach, regulates the LU and LI, and raises Qi.

UPPER JIAO
Clears LU heat, clears lung Qi constriction.

This point is famous for ankle pain. It will treat the entire ankle, but it is best for ankle pain that is on the yin channels.

REACTION AREA
Lung, Heart

LOCATION AND NEEDLE TECHNIQUE
Located on the LU channel, at the side of the first metacarpal bone and at the junction of the white and red skin. The needle is angled from the base of the distal thumb joint, towards PC 7. This is a superficial needle insertion. If you pull up the skin a bit, it will allow the needle to glide from the thumb joint base toward PC 7. I use a 1.5 cun needle to cover the entire area. This is not a painful point. It only hurts if you insert the needle incorrectly.

Xiao Jie

CLASSICAL INDICATIONS
Ankle pain

CLINICAL APPLICATIONS
This point is very close to 22.01 and 22.02, and thus includes some indications of those points such as neck pain and upper neck issues. This point was made popular and is used a lot to treat ankle pain and digestive issues, because it goes through the area of LU 10, the fishes belly. Because of the image and channel relationships, it is clinically effective to treat the ankle, shoulder, neck, and back.

Because of its relationship with the LU and LI, there are indications for chest pain related to the LU, general stomach problems, LI issues, and chronic weak stomach and spleen Qi.

RESOURCES

Brad Whisnant and Deborah Bleecker can be reached at:

masteringtungacupuncture@yahoo.com

www.sthelensacupuncturist.com

www.masteringtungacupuncture.com

Please sign up for our mailing list to be notified of new books and training sessions.

REFERENCES

Practical Atlas of Tung's Acupuncture – 2014
Henry McCann and Hans-Georg Ross

Lectures on Tung's Acupuncture – Points Study, 2008
Tung's Acupuncture, 2005
Lectures on Tung's Acupuncture Therapeutic System, 2008
Dr. Wei Chieh Young

Acupuncture 1, 2, 3
Dr. Tan's Strategy of 12 Magical Points
Twelve & Twelve in Acupuncture
Twenty-Four More in Acupuncture
Richard Teh-Fu Tan and Stephen Rush, OMD, LAc.

Introduction to Tung's Acupuncture – 2014
Dr. Chuan-Min Wang DC L.Ac. (Author), Steven Vasilakis LAc (Editor)

Advanced Tung Style Acupuncture: The Dao Ma Needling Technique of Master Tung Ching Chang
James H. Maher

Master Tung's Acupuncture: An Ancient Alternative Style in Modern Clinical Practice, Oct 1992
Miriam Lee

Jing Jin: Acupuncture Treatment of the Muscular System using the Meridian Sinews– 2010
David Legge

The Yellow Emperor's Classic of Medicine: A New Translation of the Neijing Suwen with Commentary– May 10, 1995
Maoshing Ni

Dao of Chinese Medicine: Understanding an Ancient Healing Art– August 15, 2002
Donald Edward Kendall

Mapping the Mind– August 18, 2010
Rita Carter

A Manual of Neuro-Anatomical Acupuncture, Volume I: Musculo-Skeletal Disorders– January 1, 1999
Joseph Y. Wong

Fundamentals of Chinese Acupuncture (Paradigm title)– February 1991
Andrew Ellis, Nigel Wiseman, Ken Boss

INDEX

OTHER BOOKS BY BRAD WHISNANT AND DEBORAH BLEECKER

This book is part of a series of books on Master Tung and other theories of distal acupuncture. Please visit our website, www.masteringtungacupuncture.com for a complete list of books and videos on Master Tung. If you sign up for our mailing list, we will notify you about new books and seminars.

We can be reached at masteringtungacupuncture@yahoo.com.

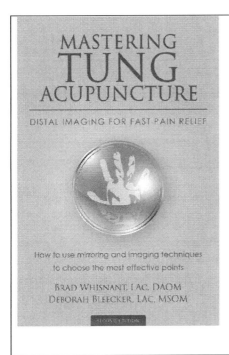

Mastering Tung Acupuncture - Distal Imaging for Fast Pain Relief, Second Edition

Learn the science behind why the image and mirror theory works to help you find the most effective distal points.

Understand how mirror images apply to Master Tung and TCM points. Letters to Brad section includes 18 letters answering questions on distal acupuncture, and how to treat complicated ailments.

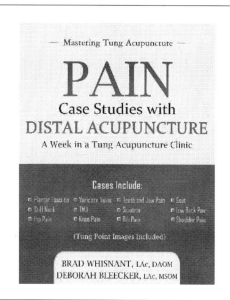

Pain Case Studies with Distal Acupuncture: A Week in a Tung Acupuncture Clinic

** All New Tung Point Images in each case study.

Cases include Back Pain, Plantar Fasciitis, Neck Pain, Stiff Neck, Trigger Finger, Hip Pain, Groin Strain, Gout, Knee Pain, Teeth Pain, Varicose vein pain.

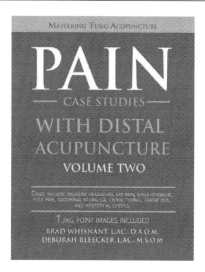

Pain Case Studies with Distal Acupuncture - Volume Two

This is the --2nd book of case studies
All new case studies.
New Tung point images for every case study

Cases include Migraine headaches, ear pain, sinus headache, foot pain, trigeminal neuralgia, carpal tunnel, interstitial cystitis, and throat pain.

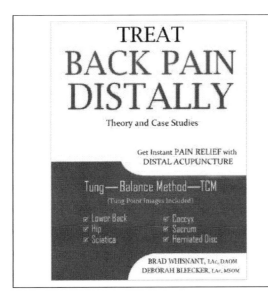

Treat Back Pain Distally
How to treat every type of lower back pain with the Balance Method and Tung points. All point images included in each case. Point locations listed in the back. Over 300 pages. Everything you wanted to know about relieving back pain with distal acupuncture. Case studies and theory included for the lower back, hip, sciatica, coccyx, sacrum pain, and how to treat a herniated disc.

This book is part of a series of books about Tung and distal acupuncture. Please check your book distributor for new book

Made in the USA
San Bernardino, CA
19 February 2016